Sequelae of Parental Separation

Ashoka Jahnavi Prasad

Copyright © 2015 Professor Ashoka Jahnavi Prasad

Institute All Rights Reserved

No part of this book may be used in any commercial manner without express permission of the author. Scholarly use of quotations must have proper attribution to the published work. This work may not be deconstructed, reverse engineered or reproduced in any other format.

Created in Switzerland

Table of Contents

ACKNOWLEDGMENT

S INTRODUCTION
Part I: FUNDAMENTAL CONCEPTS

    1. The Process of Separation, Bereavement, and Grief

    2. The Ethological Perspective

    3. Cognitive Development and the Separation Process

    4. The Life Cycle and the Separation Process

    5. The Adolescent Heritage

    6. Adult Development and Separation from the Adolescent

    -7. Parental Separation and the Variables Affecting It

    8. Case History of Wayne Marlie

    9. Discussion of Wayne Marlie's Separation from His Parents

10. Borderline Syndrome
11. Case History of Greg Davis
12. Discussion of Greg Davis's Separation from His Parents

References

Notes

ACKNOWLEDGMENTS

Writing this book has given me the opportunity to synthesize much of the learning, experiencing, and thinking I have done during and following my years of professional training. Therefore, the acknowledgments should include all those important to me in my professional development, for they all have had their influence on this book. I have been fortunate to have had too many excellent teachers to name all of them here.

I would like to thank those who spent considerable time with me working directly on the book. Dr. Marjory Follinsbee gave me important advice and criticism on Part 3. I would like to thank the three members of my doctoral dissertation committee-Drs. Mervin Freedman, Harvey Peskin, and Norbert Ralph-for their valuable contributions to this work. I wish to express my gratitude to Dr. Carl Rutt and Mr. Gary Bloom for their considerable help in revising this work from dissertation to book form and their important contribution to the additions since completion of the dissertation.

The adolescents and parents who allowed me to get to know them form the basis of this work. Without them there simply could not have been a book such as this.

I also am indebted to the secretarial staff of the Department of Psychiatry especially

Janice Nelson, for the typing of the manuscript and editorial contributions.

INTRODUCTION

The topic of this book is the separation process that parents and adolescents go through as the adolescent moves from childhood to adulthood. I have spent about seven years studying this process, and hold this subject to be quite important. I would like to share with the reader what brought me to regard the adolescent-parental separation process as so important.

My psychotherapy training began at the Royal Edinburgh Hospital. After three years there, I completed a year long attachment at the Jung Instutute. While there, I saw, for the most part, people in their twenties who were motivated to enter psychotherapy because of a loss or an anticipated loss of an important relationship.

The cultural background of my patients was extremely diverse, and the symptoms that they presented varied. However, the precipitant that brought the people into psychotherapy most often entailed a loss or an anticipated loss. Although many had long-standing problems and had thought about seeking help, it often took this type of tragedy to bring them to psychotherapy. I found that besides the other concerns these people had, the individual's personality style, and the wide variety of defenses used in defending against anxiety, an important aspect of therapy was dealing with loss.

I further found that in those who were suffering loss-whether by causes beyond their control, such as death, or by individual motivation, such as divorce-many of the symptoms and behaviors and much of the affect appeared universal. As their psychotherapist, I needed to know what had been found to be productive in helping people through such periods and what conditions made this experience a developmental one rather than a pathological one. In exploring the issues of separation with my patients, I found that those who had had a productive developmental experience while separating from their parents during adolescence appeared to have an easier time in later separations. In a sense, an individual's separation from his or her parents served as a prototype for future separations.

Seeking positive conditions for separation, I began to look for the interpersonal conditions in adolescence that made the separation from parents a positive one, as compared to those that proved to be uncomfortable experiences adding to the possibility of discomfort and pathology in future separations. It was obvious to me then, as it is now, that the relationship between parent and child has the most significant influence on the process. However, other variables appeared important; to find these, a more systematic inquiry into the adolescent-parental separation process needed to be undertaken. Fortunately, several studies being conducted at the Wright Institute provided me with opportunities for involvement in this area.

Among these studies was one that focused on the psychosocial development of high school students still living at home. These students were interviewed in groups twice a month bimonthly over a six-month period. They filled out questionnaires, were given a full battery of psychological tests and were interviewed individually at the beginning and end of the study. Another study focused on the psychosocial development of high school students living away from home for the first time, in a private school. These students were interviewed every other month on an individual and group basis for the entire school year. Students also filled out questionnaires and were given psychological tests at the beginning and end of the school year. A third study in which I was involved focused on the psychosocial development of college freshman who were living away from home for the first time. All of these students were interviewed individually at the beginning and the end of the school year; group interviews took place every three months, and many of the students also were interviewed individually every three months over the course of the two-year study. Psychological inventories and questionnaires were filled out at the beginning and the end of each school year.

As a psychotherapist, I have gained insight into adolescent-parental separation problems from a quite different frame of reference. In the past several years my clinical activity has focused primarily on the problems of adolescents facing the separation process. I have worked with adolescents and their families both while the adolescents were at home and following their move to group home facilities or their emancipation.

While investigating the conditions of separation that seemed most beneficial, I felt that it would also be valuable to find out how other cultures have dealt with these issues. Specifically, I looked for what it was in our culture that might be contributing to turmoil or to the destructiveness of the experience for some; that is, what cultural needs appeared at odds with the individual's needs. These factors were found to have a great deal of significance. In attempting to interrelate the observations of complex material such as diverse cultural norms, diverse interpersonal relations, and recurring behavior and affect in individuals, I have found it useful to use ethological principles.

Ethology is uniquely valuable for such a task, for it allows one to interrelate such material in a meaningful way. An ethological perspective is used in this book to bring together the influences of cognition, interpersonal experience, family systems, and culture on the process of separation of parent and adolescent.

Part I of the book will begin with a summary of the major issues of interpersonal separation, grief, and bereavement. Following this will be a discussion of how the ethological frame of reference has contributed to my understanding of the separation process. The remainder of Part I will focus on the effect of cognitive development on separation, separation in the context of the life cycle, and cultural influences on separations. With this theoretical background as a basis, the adolescent-parental separation process in contemporary American middle-class society will be discussed in Part II. Through the use of case histories, a healthy developmental separation will be compared to one fraught with pain and the constriction of personal growth (Part III).

Part IV will focus on therapeutic intervention in those separation processes that have become stuck or unduly painful.

Part I
Fundamental Concepts

CHAPTER 1

The Process of Separation, Bereavement, and Grief

Although adolescent-parental separation is a natural course of the life cycle, there is a close correlation of this process to bereavement, mourning, and grief. Indeed, in many cultures the puberty rites are symbolized by death and rebirth. For example, the Australian aborigines symbolize entrance into adulthood by digging a grave which the child enters for a period. Upon emerging, the child is pronounced an adult.

Before discussing the adolescent separation, it will be valuable to review some of the major studies of the separation process.

Major Studies of the Separation Process

Charles Darwin was the first to suggest that there was universal grief reaction in humans. He based this on his observation of a similar body language response to the loss of a close associate. For example, Darwin observed that people's initial reaction to grief is an excited state including frantic movement and wringing of the hands. This is followed later by a lack of movement, obliquity of the eyebrows, and a downward turn of the corners of the mouth. This expression of grief, Darwin found, was the same regardless of cultural influence. He therefore postulated that the reaction was an innate one (Darwin 1872).

Freud, in his studies of the bereaved, found that they shared a common pattern of response to their loss. In "Mourning and Melancholia," Freud (1917) states that in both mourning, a normal reaction to loss, and melancholia, a pathological reaction to loss, there is a similar process, with one exception. The similarity includes a period of painful feelings of dejection, apathy toward the outside world, loss of capacity to love, and disinterest in activity. In the case of melancholia, he finds that the feature that distinguishes it from mourning is a lowering of self-regard, which usually entails much self reproach. Freud sees the process of both mourning and melancholia as one in which the libido needs to be withdrawn from the love object that is now gone. This is objected to by the parts of the individual that received gratification from the love object. The process, Freud states, is carried out bit by bit. Reality testing slowly shows the ego, both conscious and unconscious, that the object is no longer there and that the libido has to be withdrawn from it. Freud states that, in certain cases, mania results from this process when the libido is freed from the love object too quickly. The libido goes wild because it no longer is attached to the love object and therefore has no structuring or direction.

Freud states that both mourning and melancholia pass in time. The difference between the two is the disturbance in self-regard that increases the individual's pain and suffering in the case of melancholia. Freud goes on to say that melancholia results from the loss of a narcissistic object choice. That is, when an ego separation has not been made prior to the loss of the love object, the loss causes severe disturbance in self-regard. The attachment in such a case is symbiotic, and the love object is seen as an egocentric extension of the individual. That the object was lost becomes the responsibility of the individual, who thus must accept the guilt. This, in turn, leads to the disturbance in self-regard. Freud states that the mourning ends when the libido is withdrawn from the love object and when an alternative is found for libidinal energy. This can be either a new love object or an attachment to an internalized representative of the love object, which can occur when the person performs for himself or herself the gratification formerly received from the love object. In the latter case the person identifies with the lost object (Freud 1921, 1932).

Bowlby (1961, 1973) has studied grief reaction in children and, based on his findings and those of colleagues studying "loss" in adults, has concluded that, indeed, the grief reaction is a universal response to loss with cross-culturally shared characteristics. In his article "Childhood Mourning and Its Implications for Psychiatry," Bowlby (1961) points out that in viewing separations that go on in the life of individuals, it appears that there is a similar process that goes on in all separations, whether it be bereavement for a lost love or a child's bereavement at being separated from his parents. Even the loss of a part of the body, such as a limb, entails a similar bereavement process.

Bowlby (1973) describes three stages that he sees essentially the same for all separations, even though he developed these stages in reference to the children he observed after they had been separated from their parents. They are, namely, the stages of protest, despair, and detachment. The stage of protest in the child is characterized by tears, anger, and other behaviors that are aimed at the goal of reattachment-the primary goal of the protest stage. The second stage is that of despair. Its goal is the coming to terms with the reality of the separation. This stage is characterized in the child by his being sad, distant, and unresponsive. At times there are regressions back to activities such as those seen in the protest stage, but these are usually for brief periods only. The final stage is that of detachment. During this stage the child moves from a depressed affect and lack of interest in other people to an attenuation of the attachment feelings, the return of activity, and an openness to new relationships. During the final stage, the child may at times have brief periods of sadness and grief characteristic of the earlier ones; however, they become less and less evident in this stage as the attenuation becomes more pronounced. Prior to the third stage, if the parents were to return, the child would be as attached as ever. The third stage marks the gradual attenuation of the relationship, so that if the parents return, the child will no longer be as attached.

Bowlby sees the behaviors in the initial two stages as having the goal of maintaining the attachment relationship. The effect of the child's behavior on parents in the first stages discourages further separation. The behaviors in the third stage, however, are aimed at giving the child the best chance of surviving without the attachment. A successful completion of the process of mourning for the child entails a new attachment to a new adult parental figure. Bowlby states that the following attachment may never be as strong as the original. This, however, depends on factors such as age and quality of the preceding attachment. The one major difference between separation in childhood and that in later life is the child's greater need to form a new attachment as part of the final stage of the separation process. One reason for this may be that identification with the lost object is an important part of separation resolution. The young child is unable to do this, however, since, as will be discussed further on, identification entails formal operations cognition for object relations to be fully internalized. It also is of survival value for a child to form a new attachment immediately. With this exception the stages of separation in children are similar to the separation processes of adults.

In his studies of bereavement in adults, Parkes (1972) reports the results of his study of bereavement in widows and widowers in London.[1]

Parkes divided the process of bereavement into five stages, which overall closely correspond to Bowlby's three stages. Parkes refers to the first stage of bereavement as "alarm," which is a reaction to the loss characterized by a generalized fear response. There is a strong sympathetic nervous system response, general restlessness, and a feeling of danger. This is not directed at the lost object, however; it is a directionless response. In this stage of grief there is pervasive disbelief that the loss has occurred.

The first stage passes quickly. The person then enters the second stage, which Parkes calls "searching." There is an outward acceptance of the loss now. In this stage there are episodic pangs of grief that become rather acute and that are similar to the alarm stage. There is no prolonged depression, but there remain an inner disbelief that the love object is gone and a feeling of wanting to search for it. There is, furthermore, a sense of being incomplete, or identity diffusion. The person in this stage often seems to avoid any reminders of the lost person. Descriptions of feelings during this period often include that of being pulled in two directions- avoidance and search.

This leads into the third stage, called "mitigation." It is characterized by a general feeling that the love object is nearby, although he or she cannot be seen or heard. Parkes found that widows and widowers would often talk to the lost person during this period and that they had frequent episodes of pining and feelings of nostalgia. At other times, they would completely put the loss out of their minds, using defenses of denial to avoid all reminders of the past.

In this period, the individual's conscious reality testing is working to prove the loss to the side of the person that does not want to believe that there is a loss. This ambivalence results in an oscillation between shutting out reminders of the loss and embracing reminders that the love object is gone. The danger in this stage is that if the person had been overly dependent on the love object, it may be too difficult for him or her to work through the loss. Parkes describes this stage as having three main components: preoccupation with memories of the person; painful, repetitious recollections of the loss experience, which continue until the loss is accepted; and an attempt to make sense of the loss, that is, to give it a life meaning. Philosophy, religion, and creative activity often come into play in this stage of mourning, as the person sees his or her world in chaos and works to give it some kind of order. This stage ends with a true acceptance of the loss, on both a conscious and an unconscious level. This frees the strong affectual response to the loss.

Parkes calls the fourth stage "anger and guilt," which includes depressive withdrawal. The feelings of apathy and a depressive mood are much different from the pangs of depression felt in earlier stages. This depression is described by the bereaved as a dull, withdrawn feeling of sadness and despair. During this period, feelings of guilt come to the forefront, since all relationships involve some degree of ambivalence. How this guilt is dealt with may have a significant effect on whether or not pathological mourning develops.

When the loss is successfully faced on an affectual level, the fifth stage begins. With the reality of the loss rationally and affectively incorporated, the individual is free to reintegrate his or her identity, separate from the lost object. In doing this, the bereaved must learn to do for himself or herself those things for which he had formerly depended on the other person. This includes both psychic and physical gratification. This stage is not unlike Freud's process of identification with the lost object, but Parkes describes it in broader terms. In some instances, the bereaved introjects the strengths of the other person; in other instances, he or she seeks out similar qualities in other individuals. The beginning of this period is characterized by feeling empty and lost and by a desire to find one's self. It concludes with the establishment of a new identity.

The quality that Parkes found differentiated persons suffering atypical grief from those for whom the periods of grief and mourning proceeded in more healthy ways was the significant amount of guilt in those who became pathologically depressed. The period of grief in this group was often prolonged and delayed. Parkes, like Freud, found that if the relationship was symbiotic prior to separation, pathology was more likely. For example, hypochondriacal illnesses often developed in those people who experienced a more symbiotic form of introjection as a result of difficulties in object relations existing before the period of grief began. Another factor that contributed to variability in the amount of turmoil as a result of grief was the amount of time and preparation that was allowed the person prior to the loss. Those people who had an opportunity to begin to deal with the loss prior to its actually taking place-for example, slowly developing cancer-seemed to be able to get through the bereavement period less painfully. Possibly, they were able to deal more directly with their feelings of guilt with the person while he or she was still alive. Furthermore, their life probably changed more gradually, allowing them more time to find new meaning in new things. This is somewhat similar to the anthropological conclusions to be discussed regarding adolescent transition-that is, the more gradual the process, the less stressful. It is also interesting to note that Parkes did a study of adults who lost limbs and found that their responses to the loss included stages of grief that were very similar to the stages that widows and widowers went through.

Edelson discusses the separation process from the perspective of the intensely close relationship of analyst and patient involved in longterm, intensive psychotherapy. Edelson states that the major issue in termination of psychotherapy is that in the pain of separation man is confronted with the impermanence of his own condition, the insecurity derived from the realization of his impermanence, and the impermanence of his environment. In the termination of psychotherapy, all the issues that are bound up in past separations, in past transitions, and in past losses are reflected and reviewed. He states that because it is an opportunity to review past losses, it is, therefore, a painful experience.

There are three major themes in the process of termination in therapy, which Edelson divides into stages. The first stage, "a response to the narcissistic wound," includes panic, rage, a pervasive sense of worthlessness, and a loss of wholeness. The second stage includes the theme of mourning, with accompanying feelings of guilt and grief. The third stage entails the theme of struggle toward maturity and independence, including feelings of competiveness, defiance, envy, jealousy, and the anxiety associated with these.

The first stage-the response to the narcissistic wound-includes issues of oral deprivation, basic trust, feelings of being controlled, panic, rage, and a perception of omnipotence in both the therapist and the self. He states that ideally there is an eventual recognition that neither the patient nor the therapist is omnipotent-that they face, as equals, the difficulties of the human experience. He points out, however, that it is toward the end of the first stage of mourning before the patient can tolerate seeing the therapist realistically. With the realistic view of the therapist accepted, the termination process comes to the end of the first stage.

The second stage of mourning entails facing the feelings of sadness and grief associated with the separation. Edelson states that some patients attempt to destroy any remembrance of the therapist in order to avoid the grief. Suicidal fantasy and acting out sometimes occur. Whereas the first stage dealt primarily with the intellectual acceptance of the separation, this stage is concerned with an affectual acceptance.

The final stage entails a struggle for maturity and independence. Edelson believes that at first this struggle comes out of a desire to please the therapist-to prevent losing him or her. Later, it comes out of a desire to provide for oneself what the therapist had provided, with an ensuing identification process. An internalization of the therapist's strengths provides a greater feeling of self-confidence and self-worth. Edelson states that if patients feel that they have gotten something from therapy-that is, a stronger sense of self-they can afford to give something up, that being the therapist. One issue, he points out, is very important in this process, and it is important in adolescence as well-that is, the patient's concern "Will the therapist still care for me if I do not need him anymore?" and "Is his caring for me based on my needing him?" These feelings need to be dealt with successfully by both the patient and the therapist, so that the patient can move toward independence.

In this final period there is often an escalation of feelings of competition.

For example, patients may make their own interpretations, feeling that they are as good as or better than any interpretations the therapist may have made. This comes out of a desire to test out self-reliance and out of feelings of identification with the therapist. Patient may, in fact, begin to take control of the separation process. Edelson describes the dream of one patient experiencing this in the symbolism of the puberty rite. The patient states that in the dream he wanted to become one of the men of the tribe and knew he had to give up something to be acceptable. He had to go through a painful ordeal, a renunciation of grandiose, inflated narcissism. This was symbolized by the circumcision ceremony. The dream concluded with fantasies of outdoing the father.

> Edelson states that during termination, ambivalence-love and hate, enthusiasm and apathy, optimism and pessimism, wanting to leave and wanting to stay-becomes explicit. Patients, he states, finally make the commitment to separate from therapy, to terminate the therapy despite continued ambivalence. In successful therapy patients know they are ambivalent, yet they decide that this is a productive developmental step and therefore will terminate. During the last days of therapy, Edelson often finds the patients depressed, feeling lonely, and yet wanting to go through with the termination. He states that it is very important to allow for future communication, even after a date for termination has been set and therapy completed. This is because patients should not see termination as an absolute

cutoff point; they do have a way back if absolutely necessary. The therapist does not usually expect patients to return, but it is essential that patients understand that they are not being rejected. Edelson also makes the point that in termination, therapists experience some of the same feelings as their patients and have to watch themselves so that their countertransference does not contribute to the anxiety and guilt of the patient.

One obvious significant difference between termination in psychotherapy as described by Edelson and that in bereavement as described by Parkes is that there is a way back to the therapist if necessary. In other words, the patient has some sense of choice. Although the separation process is similar, the ability to feel choice is an important variable. The bereavement process is usually much more traumatic for this reason. In discussing adolescents leaving parents, the importance of this variable will be evident in the difference between adolescents leaving home as a maturational development and those being rejected by parents. Those being rejected face the same lack of choice, that is, trauma, as Parkes' bereaved. Although separation as a result of divorce will not be dealt with here, it has been described as having a process similar to that of the other separations already described (Weiss 1975).

Recurring Themes in Separation Studies

The initial response to separation is an attempt to reattach and a feeling of being injured. This may include protestations, alarm, panic, fear, and hyperactivity. The affect is not directed, but free-floating. There are also a general sense of identity diffusion and an apathetic attitude toward new relationships, which last until the bereavement period is at least somewhat resolved. As the panic subsides, there are a disbelief that the object is lost and a desire to search for it. When reattachment attempts fail, the individual must grapple with the reality of the loss. This is done by alternately embracing memories of the lost object and feeling overwhelmed by these feelings and avoiding the memories. When the loss is intellectually accepted, the issue becomes one of coming to terms with it on an affectual level. This entails what we commonly refer to as depression and despair. During the stage of separation, the individual embraces the feelings that were a part of the relationship and withdraws from them gradually. As ambivalence is involved in all close relationships, feelings of anger and guilt become evident in this period.

When the affect has been confronted, the person, by the process of identification and internalization of his or her most important qualities, gives up the attachment.

There was a good deal of consensus that guilt-that is, a disturbance in self-regard from anger at oneself, resulting from highly ambivalent feelings within the relationship-tended to make it more likely pathological experience. There was also general agreement that the more gradual the separation, the less stressful. A symbiotic relationship is the most difficult from which to withdraw.

There are some factors in the adolescent-parental separation process that differ from those previously discussed. Adolescent-parental separation is a natural part of the life cycle. It is initiated by development in capabilities for self-sufficiency, cognition, and the desire for independence. It is encouraged by the culture, especially the peer group that shares in the experience.

This separation process is also different in that it is not the complete disengagement of the relationship, but is a change from a child-parent relationship to a more equal or symmetrical adult-to-adult relationship. However, in order to make this change, many needs that were previously fulfilled by the relationship must be withdrawn before other modes of relating can be established. In essence, certain expectations, modes of response, and fulfillments must die. The powerful child-parent relationship so necessary to child development must now die in order to allow the young adult to pursue independently his or her future.

Facing the death of the child-parent relationship is a bereavement process indeed, and it includes essentially the same major tasks that must be faced by all those who grieve. This process, as with all bereavement processes, can be a mild response or a powerful, overwhelming one; it can be a developmental experience or a constricting one. The variables affecting this process will be discussed in subsequent chapters.

Stages of Bereavement as Applied to the Child-Parent Relationship

Stage 1. The first stage is *the control of the impulse to remain attached.* The motivation for separation is highly ambivalent, and in order for the process to begin, the control over the part of the individual that wants to remain attached must be gained. Further, the adolescent feels a diffusion of his former childhood identity, and this identity diffusion remains until the separation has been completed. Likewise for the parents there is an identity diffusion as they are facing the prospect of no longer being needed by the adolescent.

The imagery that can be associated with this stage is the adolescent and parent holding onto each other with one hand, while pushing as hard as possible with the other. Once the impulse to remain attached has been at least partially controlled, the next stage begins.

Stage 2. The major issue of this stage is *cognitive realization of the separation,* the proving to the self, parents, and world that the separation has taken place. This often entails taking increasing financial responsibility, greater temporal and spacial separation, and, most important, more independence in decision making. In some instances it may also entail testing belief systems different from those of the parents and testing limits of selfreliance and self-control. As with the other separation processes, the major task of this stage is to prove to the ego that there is a separation. When the individual gains an existential sense that he or she is gaining some separation, the next stage begins.

Stage 3. This stage relates to *the affective response to the separation.* As with the other separation processes, for the adolescent and parent this entails working through depression, ambivalence, and associated guilt. Furthermore, as in the previously discussed separations, there is a desire to make sense of the separation and of its associated affects. The way in which ambivalence and guilt have been previously handled has an important impact on this task. When the affect has been somewhat worked through and mitigated, the next stage begins.

Stage 4. The adolescent, through both conscious and unconscious *identification,* undergoes internalization of the important gratifications that the child-parent relationship had previously provided and thereby begins to be able to provide these for himself or herself. When adolescents are able to provide for these needs themselves, the next stage begins.

Stage 5. In this stage, with an *attenuation of the child-parent relationship,* the door opens to a *new identity and new relationships with parents* and with others.

CHAPTER 2

The Ethological Perspective

The study of ethology began with Darwin's theory as set forth in *On the Origin of the Species by Means of Natural Selection* (1859) and, more directly, in *The Expression of Emotions in Man and Animals* (1872). (For a more comprehensive discussion of ethology, see Eibl-Eibesfeldt (1970), Breger (1974), and Bowlby (1969).) In this later work, Darwin takes up the development of behavior in animals, including man, which has evolved because it contributed to survival within the environment of genetic adaption.

At this point, man's present environment must be distinguished from the environment of his genetic adaption, for they are quite disparate. The environment of an animal's genetic adaption is one that has existed for a long enough period for its genetic code to adapt those physical and behavioral characteristics successful for survival and, conversely, to eliminate those characteristics that are distinctly disadvantageous.

It is fairly well agreed upon by modern anthropologists that man's genetic heritage was that of the hunter and gatherer. Man likely has spent more than four million years adapting to this environmental life-style. Recent anthropological studies have put the beginnings of man as a unique line divergent from that of the other higher apes about four million years ago (Washburn and Moore 1974). The causes of this divergence are believed to be the change in climate and corresponding changes in vegetation from arboreal to savanna. This, in turn, made the fruits and nuts on which the tree-dwelling apes were dependent for their survival less plentiful. The two major pressures that this brought to the primates to adapt in order to survive were a greater dependency on animal protein and a change from brachiating (twoarmed, tree-swinging) to bipedal (two-legged) locomotion. This resulted in three major changes. Namely, man began to walk upright, his brain increased greatly in size, and he adopted behaviors more appropriate to a hunting and gathering existence rather than an almost completely vegetarian one. Man's bipedal locomotion was an advantage to him because it freed the use of his hands for hunting weapons (Napier 1970; Washburn and Moore 1974).

It is a general rule of evolution that a change from a vegetarian diet to a greater dependence on animal protein leads to an increase in intelligence, since it is more difficult to capture prey than to gather food. Thus there is a rapid increase in brain size (Washburn and Lancaster 1971).

More complex communication is advantageous to the hunter as it enables greater cooperation in highly complex hunting behaviors; thus man developed language (Washburn and Lancaster 1971). The greater complexity in behavior, which was necessary to learn in order to survive, led to an even longer childhood-that is, longer dependence on adults-than the already lengthy one of our ancestral apes. Further, the change from arboreal vegetarian to the savanna hunter and gatherer brought corresponding behavioral and cultural changes (Napier 1970; Washburn and Moore 1974).

Man has been adapting to his hunting and gathering existence until, genetically speaking, a mere twenty thousand years ago, when he first began to domesticate the animals he hunted and to cultivate some of the vegetation he gathered. The amount of actual genetic change that has taken place in the last twenty thousand years is relatively small and insignificant compared to man's first three or four million years. The environment of our genetic adaption, therefore, remains that of the hunter and gatherer.

Patterns of Behavior

Past discussions of genetic heritage have often become hung up on the nature-versus-nurture argument. The trend today is a convergence of thought that takes into account the influence on behavior of both the biological potential for behaviors and the environmental influences.

One of many arguments for this view is Lorenz's discussion in *The Evolution and Modification of Behavior* (1965) which presents a strong case for viewing behavior in this integrated framework. Those who remain at either extreme of the nature-versus-nurture argument are clearly dissident from the ever-increasing tide of evidence.

Behavior, then, is influenced to varying degrees by both phylogenetic and environmental forces. Lower-order animals are most dependent on genetic determinants, and higher-order animals are most dependent on learned behaviors.

Ethologists have formulated a series of categories that describe forms of behavior that are influenced by the environment to different degrees. The categories, arranged in order of least to most environmental influence, are as follows: fixed-action patterns, internal motivating mechanisms, innate releasing mechanisms, releasers, and innate learning dispositions (EiblElbesfeldt 1970).

Fixed-action patterns are unlearned behaviors and the least alterable by the environment. In man, these behaviors exist for a brief period following birth-for example, rhythmic searching for the breast and the grasping reflex.

Internal motivating mechanisms are behaviors aimed at achieving a phylogenetically determined goal. The actual behaviors used have greater variability than a fixed-action pattern (Eibl-Eibesfeldt 1970). For example, there is internal motivation in an infant to form attachment to a mother figure. Crying, smiling, and proximity-seeking are all behaviors that are incorporated in seeking this goal. What behaviors are actually used are a response to the environment (Bowlby 1969).

There are periods within the developmental life cycle in which there is an increased sensitivity to learn in a particular area, which will last for a defined length of time. These periods are referred to as "sensitive periods." In humans, for example, the strong motivation for attachment to a mother figure lasts from approximately six months to eighteen months of age. Following this period, if there is no attachment, the motivation and sensitivity to learn attachment attenuates greatly. These sensitive periods roughly correspond to the concept of developmental stages described by many theorists, most notably Freud. Freud's stages contain much greater complexity of motivation and broader behavioral influence than those attributed to the sensitive periods by most ethologists. Psychoanalytic theory is also based on a higher order of inference. However, the concepts of sensitive periods and stages share the notion of heightened internal motivation and sensitivity to particular areas of learning for particular lengths of time and are aimed at developmental goals.

Innate releasing mechanisms are unlearned behaviors aimed at communication with other members of the species, who reciprocate with an appropriate behavior. The smiling and crying responses are releasing mechanisms between mother and child. (Deaf and blind children smile and cry.) Many of these behaviors, although altered by experience, remain throughout the life cycle (Eibl-Eibesfeldt 1970; Hass 1972).

Releaser is the term applied to expressive movements and other social signals. These are important throughout life and can be altered by experience. Kissing can serve as a sexual releaser leading to necking, which can, in turn, lead to seeking horizontal posture, leading to more direct tactile stimulation of sexual organs, which can lead to intercourse. However, the behavior can take on different meanings and can be terminated at any point.

Innate learning disposition refers to a propensity to learn and to behaviors that encourage learning in certain areas. For example, man has a strong propensity to learn to speak. Human infants are the most innately verbal of all primates and, of course, all animals. Babies are constantly babbling and, as they grow older, tend to mimic the sounds they hear with increasing frequency; this ultimately leads to the development of speech. In man the innate disposition to learn remains a strong influence on his behavior throughout life (Eibl-Eibesfeldt 1970).

In the evolution from the earliest primates to great apes to man, there has been an ever-increasing dependency on learned behavior, with a corresponding attenuation of genetic influence. For man, learning has become so important it can, at times, completely overshadow genetic influences on behavior. This capacity can have tremendous survival advantages to the species but can also be a liability. The advantage of learning abilities to one's survival potential is that they allow quicker adaptation to a more diverse environment and to a changing environment. The greater reliance on learned behavior, however, increased the potential to stray further from behavior related to survival, bringing about a greater potential for self-destructive behavior.

Indeed, man has the greatest potential for pathological or selfdestructive behavior. From the individual's point of view, however, he is often in a desperate search for those behaviors he hopes will be most beneficial to him when he is being most self-destructive. For example, even a suicidal person is not seeking his self-destruction, but the removal of psychic pain.

Ethology and Human Behavior

Bowlby (1969) has developed a theoretical construct for applying ethological principles to the study of human behavior that has been found useful in investigating adolescent-parental separation.

Borrowing from Wiener (1948), Bowlby analogizes the course of man's behavioral modes to that of a guided missile seeking a target in what he calls a "control systems approach." As a guided missile heads toward its target, it continually receives feedback on its progress. If it has roved from its target's direction, it uses this feedback to readjust its direction until it is consistent with its path. The end goal for man is the survival of the human race, and there are corresponding subgoals that must be met for the overall goal of survival. (These subgoals are not unlike Murray's [1938] concept of needs or Bateson's [1972] concept of homeostatic mechanisms.) For example, he must eat, find a mate, and raise his young. These goals, in turn, have subgoals. The individual proceeds toward these goals, while receiving constant feedback as to how he is progressing. If he is straying from the direction of his goal, he corrects his behavior, bringing his course into greater compliance with the goal.

Man starts out his journey with a variety of subgoals, such as eating and security, and a limited number of behaviors for achieving these ends (for example, crying, sucking, and smiling). As he gets older, more subgoals are added, the feedback system becomes more complex, and the repertoire of corrective behaviors grows. Along with these changes, the internalized map (our cognitive process) that views and gives feedback on the progress toward the goals becomes increasingly more complex as the child matures.

The basic elements of the process of adolescent separation as set forth in this book do not necessarily stand on the principles of ethology alone - they are closely tied to observable behaviors. What the ethological perspective has provided is a map to the interrelatedness of behaviors that heretofore have not been seen as interrelated. One of the outcomes of viewing human development with the benefit of the ethological map is the ability to reassess the interrelatedness of the separation process, the identification process and the process of a child's development of morality and life goals, or what Freud referred to as "superego." Heretofore, this process has been discussed primarily from a psychoanalytic view. The following discussion, based on an ethological perspective, provides new insight into the interrelationship of these developmental processes.

A Reassessment of the Identification Process and Its Relationship to the Separation Process

Freud (1921, 1932) discussed the process of primary identification, in relationship to the resolution of the Oedipal complex, as a way in which the child dealt with ambivalence of carnal desire for the mother and fear of the father. Although some of Freud's observations regarding identification appear correct-that is, the child at the "Oedipal" ages does incorporate many of his father's characteristics-the inference that it is a result of competition does not necessarily follow. The conflict of interests that Freud refers to in the Oedipal complex may certainly be an addition to the general ambivalence of a child's movement toward greater autonomy. However, as Sanford (1967) points out, Freud's concept of identification as part of the Oedipal conflict leaves unexplained much of a child's motivation to acquire parental traits. Those who have tried to build on Freud's original theory still have not satisfactorily explained the process. For example, the resolution of the Oedipal complex as well as the resultant identification with the agressor, is alleged to be the heir to the superego. This leaves unexplained the strong superego of one-parent children. Bowlby and Paris have suggested that many of the issues that Freud saw as Oedipal were, in fact, issues of separation-individuation. Bowlby has done a reinterperation of Freud's case of "Little Hans," in which he redefines the conflicts experienced by Hans as related to issues of separation rather than Oedipal issues (Bowlby 1973). In his reexamination, Paris (1976) concluded that the issues Freud referred to in the Oedipal complex can be interpreted as resulting from a number of developmental sources but, most important, separation-individuation issues. As Bowlby (1969) and Averill (1968) point out, separation is difficult, and, from an ethological perspective, it is meant to be, because group cohesiveness for both the child and the adult of the hunting and gathering group was essential to survival.

The initial motivating mechanisms are, therefore, aimed at discouraging separation. When this fails, mechanisms in the later stages of separation are aimed at making the individual more likely to survive without the lost relationship. For the child this entails reattachment. For the adult it entails an ability to provide for oneself, both psychologically and physically, that which had been previously provided by the departed person. This entails mechanisms that promote identification with the departed person in the later stages of the separation process. Identification here refers to the individual qualities that are valuable and rewarding being internalized by both conscious and unconscious processes. This internalization includes the necessary elements of socialization, that is, the superego.

This ethological perspective of the separation process contradicts psychoanalysis with regard to the question of identification. In the psychoanalytic view, the major mover of identification is the Oedipal complex, identification with an aggressor. However, evidence supports the separation process as being the primary motivation for identification.

The development of inherent competition between father and son or mother and daughter could only occur, according to the ethological principle, if there were survival advantages involved or at least an absence of a negative effect on survival. Throughout evolution there has, in fact, been a clear absence of competition between offspring and parent during the young's development, because this would be clearly injurious to the survival chances of the species. On the other hand, a process whereby the young have a propensity to copy what is valuable in the older generation would have a clear survival advantage for the species. This is essentially what happens in the separation process.

The interrelationship of separation and identification is not a new concept. Levinson (1970) writes as follows with regard to the termination of a mentor-protégé relationship:

> The younger man, in turn, feels appreciation, admiration, respect, gratitude, love, and identification. The relationship is lovely for a time, then ends in separation arising from a quarrel, death, or change in circumstances. Following the separation the process of internalization is enhanced, since internalization is increased by loss and the personality of the mentee is enriched as he makes the valued qualities of the mentor more fully a part of himself. In some respects the main value of the relationship is created after it ends, but only if there is something there when it is happening. This is probably true of psychotherapy as well (pp. 251-252).

These observations strongly support identification as primarily motivated by the separation process rather than the Oedipal complex.

CHAPTER 3

Cognitive Development and the Separation Process

Cognitive development is an important influence on the separation process. There are cognitive capacities that must be developed before attachment between mother and child can occur. Following this there must be cognitive changes that allow the child to move toward greater autonomy. Poorly developed cognitive functioning can greatly inhibit the separation process.

The two most important aspects of cognition's influence on separation are the cognitive modes of response to change-namely, what Piaget refers to as assimilation and accommodation-and the movement toward everincreasing complexity in the abstract cognition of object constancy (Piaget and Inhelder 1969). In conceptualizing his findings on the development of cognition in children, Piaget has related this development to the process of evolution; he uses the biological term "assimilation" to describe the process of understanding perceptions of the world in the existing frame of reference. Piaget describes pure assimilation as being play. That is, in play children can manipulate the world they create to conform perfectly to their perceptions of it. "Accommodation" is the term he uses to describe the alteration of the individual's frame of reference in order to bring his or her perceptions and cognition into concurrence. Pure accommodation is described as imitation where the individual completely adopts a new frame of reference, abdicating his or her old one.

In a secure, but challenging, environment, an equilibrium is reached between these modes of development so that the child neither mimics those around him, nor lives in a total fantasy world. A child will use either mode of response at the expense of the other when the environment is overly complex or chaotic for the individual's stage of development, when good role models and teachers are lacking, and when it is impossible for the child to find any integrated response that is successful.

A combination of both biological capability and motivation, with a secure but stimulating environment, leads to an increasingly complex understanding of the environment. For example, I once played a table-top game of football with an eight-year-old boy. It was, according to the rules, supposed to last for four, fifteen-minute quarters. I only had thirty minutes free, so I suggested that we play two, fifteen-minute halves. To this lad, the rules were God-given, and we could play either one hour or not at all. He could only assimilate the choices into his existing view of the rules, which, to him, seemed unalterable. This eight-year-old boy could not understand that the rules were by mutual agreement; in other words, he could not accommodate a new frame of reference. Through support and encouragement he agreed to try, and he found the game could be altered without destroying it. Thus, he was able to reach a new equilibrium between assimilation and accommodation.

Piaget divides cognitive development into periods or stages. The first is the sensorimotor period, in which the child learns that objects are separate from himself or herself and that they are permanent. This is usually fully accomplished when the child is about eighteen to twenty-four months of age; the period of preoperational thinking then emerges. The major cognitive task of this period is to learn to use symbols to represent the world, especially language. Concrete operations begin at about six years of age. During this period the child learns to make generalizations and categories in relating to concrete things and events. In adolescence the formal operations period begins. The adolescent develops the capacity to manipulate abstract concepts. He can hypothesize, extrapolate into the future, and introspect.

The general trend in cognitive development is a moving away from egocentrism to a greater capacity for relativistic thinking and empathy. In each stage the new capacity that is developed is, at first, egocentric and tested to extreme limits. Through the process of achieving an assimilationaccommodation equilibrium that is effective in dealing with the world, there is a decentering (Breger 1974). As an example of the development of formal operations, adolescents are able to hypothesize about the future; they often spend a good deal of time fantasizing about the utopia they expect to create. It is often very difficult for them to give up this egocentric fantasy. This perception of reality, however, soon brings adolescents into conflict with the reality of the world.

As with previous situations, this novel situation—a result of both cognitive and social development—must be dealt with by assimilation and accommodation. If adolescents' environment provides opportunities to experiment and to receive realistic feedback, they will develop satisfying, creative, and realistic goals through an integration of both assimilation and accommodation. The movement in adolescence from a child dependent on parents to the reality of adult independence is a profound cognitive challenge. In order for this to be mastered adaptively, it is essential that both modes of assimilating and accommodating the new reality are within adolescents' and parents' capability.

The area of increasingly complex cognition that is most important to the separation process is object constancy and object relations. This is initially begun at six months of age, when acquiring the capacity to realize that the mother exists as a separate entity from oneself is the major task. This cognitive ability must, then, become increasingly complex to allow for greater autonomy. For example, children must be capable of realizing that their desires and those of their mothers are not always the same, yet they still have an attachment. Further, children must be able to recognize that their behavior can bring a corresponding behavior from their mothers-for example, when the child cries, the mother comes.

As children increase their cognitive capabilities, they become able to feel safe and secure within the attachment, with increasing distance both temporally and spatially. For infants, the mother must be present for the attachment to feel secure. For fifteen-year-olds, the attachment may feel secure because they know that a telephone call to their mothers, even if two thousand miles away, can bring a sense of parental protection and security.

During adolescence, cognitive development affects the separation process in two ways. First, the adolescent's capabilities and experiences in dealing with novel situations through the modes of assimilation and accommodation will dictate how he or she deals with the novel situation of separation. Second, the development of formal operations, especially regarding the capabilities for abstracting object constancy, has a profound influence on the separation process. What must be developed in adolescence is an abstract, formal operations concept of object constancy, that is, the ability to recognize not only that objects exist apart from oneself but that people have patterns of behavior that they follow with some degree of consistency, which therefore makes them somewhat predictable. On the basis of these observations, one can know how to respond to another with some rationality. An example of this is trusting only those who have been trustworthy in the past, rather than the more immature behavior of trusting everyone or trusting no one. This more abstract form of object constancy makes possible more complex internalization of parental patterns through the identification process. If this is not developed, the internalization process remains very concrete in nature.

Erikson (1950) differentiates the levels of internalization by calling the more concrete one "introjection" and the abstract internalization level "identification." He also points up the importance of a consistent predictable relationship between mother and child to the development of this more complex cognition. He states that the mechanisms of introjection and projection which prepare the basis for later identification depend for their relative integration on the satisfactory mutuality between mothering adult and mothered child (Erikson 1950). He points out that for those whose relationship with their mother has been chaotic, developing this abstract form of object constancy can be quite difficult, and thus identification cannot adequately be accomplished.

In the preceding chapters, the importance and centrality of identification to the resolution of the bereavement process was noted. It follows, then, that the cognitive ability for adequate identification is a significant variable in the process.

Marris (1974) stresses the importance of this cognitive process beyond all others to the ultimate resolution of the bereavement process. He states:

> Once we recognize that loss cannot be made good merely by substitution, the logic of mourning becomes apparent. If life is to seem meaningful again, it is not enough that the present should still be notionally worthwhile. The bereaved must be able to identify in each concrete event they experience some response worth making. The vitality of that response depends upon a commitment of purpose, which has already been given and cannot now be wished away, even though the relationships which incorporated it have been disrupted. Hence, as I have tried to show, grief works itself out through a process of reformulation, rather than substitution. Confidence in the original commitment is restored by extracting its essential meaning and grafting it upon the present. This process involves repeated reassurances of the strength and inviolability of the original commitment, as much as a search for the terms on which reattachment would still make life worth living. Until this ambivalent testing of past and future has retrieved the thread of continuity, it is itself the only deeply meaningful activity in which the bereaved can be engaged. Conventions of mourning acknowledge this, giving form and status to grief, protecting the bereaved from demands for responsive behavior which they are not yet ready to make (p. 91).

In the adolescent-parental separation process, finding the "thread of continuity" of which Marris speaks is essentially the process of identification that has been discussed. It takes place primarily in the fourth stage of the bereavement process, occurring through assimilation and accommodation of the lost object (the parents) into the new reality of adult status. Parents will readily recognize this issue in the following example.

Mary has, from the time she was eight, regularly made her bed. She turns fourteen and her bed is seldom made. Nagging is of little use; although she hates being nagged and therefore has good reason to make her bed, she does not.

This change in behavior has several likely sources, including rebellion against parental authority and testing limits, but it also has a meaning relevant to this discussion—namely, making the bed has lost its original meaning. Mary used to make her bed because of the child's desire for parental approval, that is, to be a "good" child. To an adolescent, however, "good" is seen in broader terms; it must be redefined into the prospective of the adult. Until what is "good" and purposeful is redefined, the search is, as Marris points out, "the only deeply meaningful activity," therefore, the bed does not get made.

In the fourth stage of the separation process, Mary will work to find out what are the essential meanings of her identification with her parents and will work through a process of assimilation and accommodation to make these meanings consistent with her new adult identity. This process will be discussed in more detail in Part II. What should be grasped here is the importance of this cognitive process to the resolution of the adolescentparental separation process.

CHAPTER 4

The Life Cycle and the Separation Process

The adolescent-parental separation process will be more fully understood by describing its development in the greater context of psychosocial development.

Human development is, in one sense, a process of ever-increasing independence from parents. In its folk tales, one American Indian tribe uses the mother bear to epitomize what every mother should be. The mother bear directs all of her maternal activities toward making her cub independent of her. The moment the bear offspring is capable of self-reliance, the mother leaves it to its own resources.

In the human, childhood development has become the most complex and lengthy of any within the animal kingdom, reflecting the necessity to learn the most complex adult life-style. However, the central goals of childhood, that is, independence and self-sufficiency, remain the same.

Developmental Tasks

As the child matures, there are periods in which certain developmental tasks dominate the focus of the child and parent. These periods all contribute to healthy separation from parents, leading toward independent functioning. Humans share many of these developmental periods with their closest phylogenetic relatives, the monkeys and the apes; all human cultures have them in common. The most important of these tasks are as follows: the formation of attachment between infant and mother; the gaining of some sense of autonomy from this attachment, while still remaining secure within it; the control of impulse and the channeling of behavior into socially acceptable behavior; learning communication with other members of one's group; self-sufficiency in obtaining bodily needs; entrance into the decisionmaking process of one's group; emotional separation from parental figures; adult sexual functioning; finding a mate; and becoming a parent.

The capability of performing these tasks develops continuously from birth. However, during certain periods of life, one or more of them may be a more prominent motivating factor. As stated previously, Freud and others used the prominence of one or more of the motivating forces at certain ages as a basis for dividing development into stages, which loosely correspond to the ethological sensitive periods.

Birth is, of course, the first separation the child experiences. Rank (1973) gives the "birth trauma" unique significance as the initiator of separation anxiety. Rank's ideas concerning separation anxiety correspond highly to this discussion. However, seeing this anxiety as related to the birth trauma is troublesome on two counts. First, why would such a fear develop in the course of evolution? Anxiety is a drain on the energies of an individual; therefore, in order to develop, it must provide a valuable motivation to offset its liability. It is difficult to find survival value in lasting anxiety relating to the birth trauma. Second, as Bowlby and other researchers demonstrate, separation anxiety does not develop until the child is six months of age. Therefore Rank's stress on the importance of separation anxiety is acceptable, but his belief that it is initiated as a result of the birth trauma must be rejected.

The first developmental task for an infant is *attachment to a parental figure.* It is the prototype attachment for the individual; as Erikson (1950) points out, basic trust or mistrust develops as a result of its outcome. The cognitive ability to realize object constancy is a necessity for its development.

The next issue is *individuation-separation.* This stage emerges as a result of several interacting developments: cognitive development, greater locomotion, muscle control, and motivations such as curiosity and individuality, which come into conflict at times with the attachment motivation. As a result, during this stage children experience ambivalence, probably for the first time. Their motivation to satisfy their curiosity and individuality conflicts with their desire to remain close for parental protection.

The cognitive process interacts with physical and interpersonal maturation to manifest this conflict. Children are capable of realizing that their own desires are not always the same as those of their parents. Further, children can use past experiences as a basis for expecting a particular response-for example, when they cry, they expect their mothers to come.

In healthy situations, a dynamic compromise is reached where the child can realize that the attachment is safe with increasing distance, both spatially and temporally. As Erikson (1950, p. 252) states, "outer control at this point must be firmly reassuring" for comfortable autonomy to develop.

Mahler (1968, 1975) emphasizes that this period is the most important in enabling the child to deal in later life, particularly in adolescence, with separation in a healthy way. She points out that if mothers are unable to separate their needs from their children's needs, a symbiotic relationship develops in which the children will not be able to separate their needs from their mothers' needs. A disturbance in object constancy follows in which children are unable to define themselves as separate from their mothers.

> If the mother withdraws her support too quickly for the child's dependency needs to be felt secure, the child's movement toward greater independence will again be stifled. The ambivalence that the child feels will

be viewed as dangerous, leading to rejection by the individual to whom the ambivalence is directed. "Splitting" is used as a defense mechanism against anxiety resulting from ambivalence. Mahler (1968) points out that individuals faced with ambivalence feel unable to cope with it and therefore project it as two split feelings: one person is seen as all-giving, while another is seen as allrejecting. Likewise, an action is viewed as either all good or all bad. Conscious awareness of ambivalence simply cannot be tolerated.

When outer control is firm, consistent, reassuring, and reflective of the child's capacity for independence, a dynamic compromise is reached. The child feels safe in the attachment with ever-increasing distance, both spatially and temporally. This task of increasing independence, which begins at eighteen months, will remain an important dynamic until separation is complete. The way it is initially handled from eighteen to thirty-six months, Mahler states, will be of the greatest importance when it becomes a central issue in adolescence.

The next issue is that of *impulse control and the ability to channel impulse into socially acceptable behavior.* The parents must teach the child to control impulses without resorting to harsh sanctions or oppressive guilt if later difficulty is to be avoided (Erikson 1950; Breger 1974). The separation process is later influenced by the nature of this training. The separation entails strong feelings of ambivalence, fear, and anger. If these are to be confronted successfully, adolescents must feel confident of controlling their impulses, especially their fear of losing control of their anger. Furthermore, adolescents' self-imposed sanctions, used to control these impulses will reflect those controls used by their parents in the adolescents' early development. If the parents are harshly punitive, the adolescents will be harshly punitive, either toward themselves or in a projected form, such as paranoia or prejudice.

Children learn how to deal with novel situations and practice increasingly complex behavior through imitation, play, and apprenticeship with an increasing range of significant others, including parental surrogates, teachers, and peers. The influence of this expanding group, especially peers, is profound during the adolescent separation. It influences identity, pressures or supports independence from the parents, and, most important, provides an opportunity to practice increasing independence (Breger 1974).

In adolescence, four interrelated issues become central: (1) formal operational thinking, with its corresponding moral development; (2) physiological maturation and its corresponding heterosexual motivation; (3) separation from parents; and (4) the emergence of adult identity.

By the time children are twelve or thirteen, they have become expert at dealing with the issues of childhood. At pubescence, they feel torn between the autonomy and esteem of adulthood and the security and lack of responsibility of childhood. They must, to become adults, also give up some of the attachment to their parents; their destinies no longer will be tied. Separation is a mutual experience for adolescent and parent-both have to deal with the ambivalences and rewards of letting go.

Eventually, adolescents move toward separation and adulthood. They are motivated and supported by biological propensity, peer support, cultural validation, and, it is hoped, parental encouragement. Without their realizing it, the separation process begins. How they deal with this stressful process will be highly influenced by how the previous developmental tasks have been accomplished.

Adolescent-parent separation is the first separation experience that is undergone with fully developed cognition and cultural awareness as well as the influence of personal development. It is in this sense the prototypic separation of life; that is, it serves as a model for future separation. As will be discussed later, it is the single most profound influence on the way in which adolescents separate from their own children. Separation from parents also seems to serve as the prototype for the separation process involved if the person experiences a divorce or the death of a loved one.

CHAPTER 5

The Adolescent Heritage

Chimpanzees are man's closest living phylogenetic relatives. Goodall (1971) points out that adolescence in man has a number of characteristics in common with that in chimpanzees. However, man has changed a great deal over the last ten million years since our line of descent parted ways with that of the chimpanzee (Washburn and Moore 1974). One must, therefore, be cautious of the temptation to anthropomorphize. Observations of chimpanzees can serve only as clues to man's genetic heritage, such as clues uncovered by anthropologists into our history of tool making. If this cautionary note is kept in mind, Goodall's sensitive and rich observations of chimpanzee adolescence provide us with some valuable clues into our own adolescent heritage. The following account is based primarily on her observations during her years at the Gombe Stream Reserve.

(Adolescence in Chimpanzees)

When the male chimpanzees reach puberty, around seven years of age, they weighed only about half of their fully mature weight of one hundred pounds. The adolescent, therefore, could not really compete in the male hierarchy for another six years, when it would finally reach its mature weight.

When the male reached pubescence, he began to be regarded as a potential challenger in the social hierarchy and therefore exercised caution when in the adult males' presence. Besides having to be more cautious, the male had to continue to spend much of his time around his mother. Goodall (1974) observed that when the adult males saw the adolescent around his mother, they tended to respond to him more as a child or juvenile than as an adult competitor. Hence, the adolescent gained some temporary relief from this social pressure.

This behavior was, however, related to how tolerant the mother was of the adolescent's presence. Some mother chimpanzees started rejecting their adolescent offspring rather early. These mothers rejected the adolescents because they did not feel comfortable with them once they, too, began to view them as adults. The more comfortable and tolerant mothers allowed their adolescents to stay with them and, to some degree, protected them from the ranking males. When their adolescents were attacked, the tolerant mothers would run up to the adult male with placating gestures, calming and distracting him from their offspring. The adolescents would, in turn, sometimes protect their mothers from other adolescents, or from females who may have been higher ranking. The alliance could be beneficial for both, if the mothers encouraged it.

Since it was too dangerous to go close to the adult males, they spent a good deal of time alone, much more than at any other time in their lives. The adult males spent most of their time grooming each other and feeding in the same vicinity. The adolescent was eager to join them, but fearful. He often compromised by sitting in sight of the adult males, watching them as they went through their daily activity. Sometimes the adolescent became so frustrated by his approach-avoidance ambivalence that he spontaneously began running from the adult males, imitating the confrontation gestures normally associated with dominance challenges among males, but doing it at a safe and increasing distance. During this time of life, according to Goodall, the adolescent male seemed to desire a great deal of reassurance from the adult males, especially after he was rebuffed. The reassuring gesture consisted of either a pat on the back or a squeeze of the hand. After being attacked, the adolescent would often risk being attacked again, coming close to the male with submissive gestures to get this reassurance. Goodall's interpretation of this behavior was that the adolescent male needs very badly to be accepted by the adult males.

To Goodall (1971), the motivation for this seems much greater in adolescence than at any other time in the chimpanzees life. She also felt that the male adolescent spent time watching the adults to learn how the male social society worked. This was the first time in their lives that the adolescent males spent time around the adult males. The adolescents had spent most of their childhood around females, who were in the same general vicinity as the males but who were not close enough for clear observation. Since imitation is important to a chimpanzee's social development, this period of observation is probably essential to the development of adult behaviors.

Another important developmental process appeared to be the practicing of adult behavior in games with peers or when alone. For example, adolescents practiced dominance-submission displays. As time went on, the adolescent spent more time in even closer proximity to the adults. As he reached full maturity and size, the adolescent began to display the hierarchical gestures toward some of the lower-ranking males—the old, the young, or the weak. At first the gestures were tentative, but as the adolescent gained confidence, he made more serious challenges to the lower- ranking males and finally gained adult status.

At this time, grooming behavior was started with some of the more tolerant males. The adolescent had to be very careful in this early stage not to appear threatening to any of the higher-ranking males until his position had stabilized. Once the male had been accepted and had found a place for himself in the adult society, he began to participate in sexual activity. Prior to this, he had usually observed adult sexuality from a safe distance in the same manner in which he had observed other activities. His first attempt appeared clumsy, but he became more adept with practice. One interesting note—

Goodall

(1971) never observed a son having intercourse with his mother, although he may have had intercourse with every other adult female. This evidence supports Freud's incest taboo.

The females also reached pubescence at around seven years of age, but they did not ovulate or become sexually active until about nine years of age. At this time, the females were viewed as potential challengers in the female dominance hierarchy (the dominance hierarchies for males and females is separate in chimpanzees) and therefore had to be careful around the adult females. As a result, the adolescent females spent a lot of time traveling with their mothers if they would tolerate this behavior. As with the males, some mothers were more tolerant of this than others. The adolescent females also spent more time on the fringes of the female group. As time went on, they took increased interest in caring for the younger offspring and would often help out the mothers who would accept their help. They began showing more protective maternal behavior with the infants and children and lessened their previous play behavior. They were especially maternal with their younger siblings.

Peer group interaction was as important to the females as it was to the males, giving the youth an opportunity to practice adult behavior. The adolescent female became interested in male attention, started sexually swelling (the signal for sexual receptivity), and became sexually active at around age nine. The females exhibited a wide range of response to the beginning of sexual activity. Some females were very aggressive sexually, others were fearful, and still others seemed to be ambivalent. Goodall observed that a females' sexual behavior and attitude most closely reflected that of her mother. If her mother was anxious, she, in turn, was usually anxious. If her mother was aggressive, she usually reflected that response. Although the females became sexually active at the age of nine, none that Goodall observed gave birth before age eleven. As they started reaching sexual maturity, they began to challenge some of the other females for status in the dominance hierarchy. They became more involved in the hierarchy as they reached full strength, much as the males did. Coincidentally, they became less attached to their mothers and would soon relate to them much as they related to any other females, although some remained close friends.

Goodall found that for some chimpanzees, adolescence was a mildly stressful period, while for others it was an extremely anxious time. One of the major variables of stress for the adolescent chimpanzee was how abruptly the mother began viewing her offspring as an adult. Those mothers who early viewed the youth as an adult forced the adolescent into a more abrupt, and therefore stressful, adjustment. This was further exacerbated by the likelihood that the other adults took their cue from the mother as to how to treat the youth. If the mother treated it as a child, the others frequently followed suit, and vice versa. This observation made by Goodall of chimpanzees, correlates with observations made by anthropologists studying human cultures. That is, they have observed that those cultures in which youth must make a rapid adjustment from childhood to adulthood cause more stress for the youth than those in which the change is more gradual.

Goodall points out that for chimpanzees, the period is usually more stressful for males since they have to leave the security of their mother's side. An observation that Goodall makes that is significant to our study of human adolescent separation is that adolescence and separation in chimpanzees brings on a heightened motivation to observe, imitate, and adopt the behaviors of adults. In this process, the mother from whom the adolescent is separating has a profound influence, serving as a role model and providing a basis for what an adult-to-adult relationship should be. This is especially true for females, whose adult sexual attitude and behavior for example, reflects that of their mother. It is also important to note that those chimpanzees whose mothers were most comfortable with the separation during this period had offspring who separated in a less stressful way.

The adolescent initially appears to be ambivalent about acting as an adult. It desires adult status, but is not yet capable of competing as an adult because of its immature stature and ignorance of some of the social relations process. The adolescent then spends a number of years observing adult behavior and practicing it alone and with peers. Then, at first tentatively, it begins to participate in adult activities with those who are the weakest or the most tolerant, and it soon gains security in its adult role.

Adolescence in Hunting and Gathering Cultures

Most cultural anthropologists agree that adolescence in hunting and gathering tribes is gradual and therefore less anxiety-producing than in contemporary society. This is explained by the early age at which children begin assuming adult responsibility, the homogeneity of primitive culture as a result of slow cultural change, and the opportunity to observe and apprentice adult activity from an early age (Benedict 1961; Mead 1928, 1930; Hollingsworth 1928). Hunting and gathering cultures also offer ample opportunity to practice adult activities in games and play.

Most primitive cultures have initiation rites, and, like all cultural rituals, they symbolically deal with the issues of concern both conscious and unconscious to participants. Initiation rites ritualistically deal with the essential issues of adolescence.

The major issues dealt with in the initiation rites of hunting and gathering cultures reflect the concern of these cultures with adolescence issues. Initiation or puberty rites in hunting and gathering tribes have a good deal of similarity among cultures. The ritual is usually enacted when an individual or a group reaches pubescence or shortly thereafter, often at a similar time each year, for example, each spring.

The initiates are first separated, either singly or as a group, from the rest of the community. The rituals test the limits and strengths of the adolescents. The adolescents are instructed and tested on their ability to maintain self-control and to know the rituals and norms of the culture. During the ritual, the youths must show complete obedience to their elders. The adolescents' isolation may last days or weeks. They must demonstrate that they can take care of themselves during this period.

Some rituals act out death and rebirth themes. Many of these ceremonies include ritualized demonstrations of submission to the tribal authority. Circumcision is often a part of the male's ritual. This is followed by a symbolic demonstration of entrance into adult status. Following this ceremony, the youth is regarded as ready for adult sexual activity, marriage, and adult social status.

The main issue that the initiation or puberty rites address is the change in identity from child to adult. This is initiated in the ceremony by separating the youths from their parents. It is also an educational process ensuring that the adolescent knows and accepts the norms of the society, as well as a testing of the limits of capability and self-sufficiency, while at the same time making certain that order and continuity are kept in the society

(Muensterberger 1975).

Muensterberger (1975) points out that initiation rites act out separation from parents as the precursor to adult status. The following passage, in which Muensterberger quotes Landtman (1927) describes an initiation rite where this is particularly well dramatized (Muensterberger 1975, p. 20):

> Here, the initiate is carried by some female relatives from his mother's side to the beach where his parents wash him thoroughly and, as the Kiwai put it in pidgen English, "take away smell belong to woman." He is then returned to the parental hut where his mother lies down at the entrance and the boy walks over her, placing one foot on her abdomen. The meaning of this act is explained by the Kiwai: "What place boy came from that time he born, he finish now along that place."

Muensterberger relates the importance of identification to this ritualized separation process in hunting and gathering tribes as well as in industrialized culture. He states, "There is a great variety of similar but modified puberty rites in civilized societies. Doubtlessly, the motivation is the same. Antagonism and rivalry with the parents of the same sex must be replaced by identification."

One example of such a rite is the circumcision ceremony. In it, the phallus, universally used as a symbol of dominance (Morris 1967), is put into the hands of the medicine man to alter into its adult form, a clear demonstration of the youth's acceptance of the medicine man's authority, that is, the cultural authority. As Freud has pointed out, ambivalence toward powerful authority is dealt with by identification. Another way of saying this is that the youth, placed in a position where he must trust the shaman with a treasured part of himself, is strongly motivated to look up to the shaman and to take on his valued strengths. The fact that the adolescent is leaving his parents to become an adult especially motivates him to acquire strength. It is quite likely that the ritual evolved because of its valuable impact on the tribesman in forming adult identity. This is an example of behavior aimed at encouraging identification with parents and parental figures as a part of the adolescent's movement away from parents.

As long as the culture remains stable, the rituals are successful. However, the rituals of these tribes collapse as their environment changes, primarily because they have lost their relevance to the environment. Adolescence then becomes stressful for these people, as it is for all members of rapidly changing cultures. This is probably due to the ambivalence associated with identifying with parents in cultures undergoing quick change. Identification is much more problematic if parental traits are not considered strengths but are seen as old-fashioned. An ambivalence toward identification is created, which, in turn, makes adolescence as a whole a much more difficult period.

The propensity of adolescents to internalize adult qualities as they separate is shared by both hunting and gathering cultures and chimpanzees. This gives further support to the innateness of the process. It is also evident that in those cultures that promote the identification process throughout the child's development there is much less stress than in cultures where identification is not promoted. In contemporary American culture, for example, boys rarely see their fathers in action at work. The cultural norms in fact inhibit this observation, and there are certainly no rituals that promote identification in adolescents.

CHAPTER 6

Adult Development and Separation from the Adolescent

Up to this point, the separation process has been viewed mostly from the perspective of the adolescent. It is a powerful experience for the parents as well. The process is indeed a dynamic interaction of parent and adolescent and is in no small way influenced by the parents' attitudes toward the separation. It is revealing to find its meaning in the context of the parents' life cycles, as has been done for adolescents. Erikson's (1950) stages of generativity and ego-integrity offer an insight into these dynamics.

In Erikson's scheme the stage of generativity develops when the individual has resolved sufficiently the issues of the identity crisis and has found intimacy in a heterosexual relationship. The focus of orientation then turns toward entering into a bond with one's mate and creating a new life.

This new life is directed toward being a successful member of the next generation. Erikson sees this motivation in the wider context of the urge to be creative and productive. He finds that for most people, having children is a necessary part of the expression of generativity. Parents are dependent on their children for the focus of much of their creative orientation. As he states:

> The fashionable insistence on dramatizing the dependence of children on adults often blinds us to the dependence of the older generation on the younger one. Mature man needs to be needed, and maturity needs guidance as well as encouragement from what has been produced and what must be taken care of. Generativity, then, is primarily the concern in establishing and guiding the next generation, although there are individuals who through misfortune or because of special and genuine gifts in other directions do not apply this drive to their own offspring. And, indeed, the concept of generativity is meant to include such more popular synonyms as productivity *and* creativity *which, however, cannot replace it* (Erikson 1950, p. 266-267).

The beginning of pubescence, along with the emergence of the desire in adolescents to be independent, means, to the parent, that this focus of generativity is coming to an end and that they must find new commitments and new directions. As Stierlin, Levi, and Savord (1971) point out, they usually find themselves, in their forties or early fifties, beginning to face a decline in some of their capabilities, such as physical strength, sex drive, and reproductive capacity. The adolescent, on the other hand, is quickly moving toward the peak of his or her capability in these areas, bringing the contrasting parental declines all the more into focus.

Erikson (1950) refers to the process of coming to terms with these issues as the crisis of ego-integrity versus despair. By crisis he does not mean a disastrous event but a critical issue to be faced. Ego-integrity, Erikson (1950) points out, is found in accepting the value and completeness in what one has generated, thereby allowing oneself to give it up. Erikson goes on to state that the process of trusting the new generation to take over entails a trusting of oneself to have been a good parent in preparing the adolescent to be independent. By seeing the value and completeness of one's creations, one gains ego-integrity; if one despairs that the new generation cannot take responsibility, he or she is also despairing over not having been a good parent. Therefore, he or she is left with failure, without ego-integrity, and, ultimately, with despair. Despair over incompleteness as a parent leads only to further disgust and to attempts to hang on to that which he or she has helped generate, leading to chronic despair. Erikson goes on to state that egointegrity is not achieved without a struggle with feelings of despair; parents must evaluate and reflect upon which of their generative goals have and have not been attained. By seeing where one has failed and by despairing for it, one also sees his or her success and gains integrity from what has been accomplished. In this evaluation, Erikson (1950 1976) points out, one sees the object of his or her generativity in the context of the society and the world as a whole. It is in parents' evaluation of themselves and of their creations in this larger context that Erikson finds the development of the wisdom of old age.

Erikson (1976) sums up this process beautifully in "Reflections on the Life Cycle of Doctor Borg" in which he talks about an old man's battle to give up his attempts to control his past creations, including his son, and the despair involved in the attempts:

> Even as Borge's old age struggle against despair makes him comprehend that what he has become must not be all that he is and must not be all that he leaves behind . . . He must find, in William James's terms "his murdered self" so as to find his living one (p. 21).

Erikson's discussion of ego-integrity versus despair generally reflects the dynamics of the adolescent separation process. This process is a loss both in terms of the child leaving home and in the larger context of the parental life cycle. It means the loss of at least a part of the parental identity and generative orientation.

This shift in the parent's relationship with the child is also the main theme in Ginott's book, *Between Parent and Teenager,* in which he states:

> Letting go is the key to peaceful and meaningful coexistence between parent and teenager; as parents, our need is to be needed; as teenagers, their need is not to need us. To let go when we want to hold on requires the utmost generosity and love (Ginnot 1969, p. 111).

The parents, then, in giving up their attachment and their dependency on the child for their self-definition and sense of esteem, must undergo a process of bereavement, in which they are influenced by the variables discussed previously in relation to all separation processes. Through the process of giving up their children, they gain a sense of integrity. They are then liberated to formulate new goals and, therefore, to see themselves in a new way.

The characteristics described in the literature that distinguished parents who were able to separate in a way which allowed them to grow and to find ego-integrity from parents constricted by feelings of incompleteness and despair in general reflected the variables previously noted in relation to the separation process. For example, Offer and Offer (1975) state that parents who were able to let go were usually the ones who felt comfortable with change. They were self-confident, had good interpersonal relationships, and were able to learn from their adolescents. Similarly Murphy et al. (1962) said that parents who had the easiest time separating shared certain characteristics, including the following:

• Being able to satisfy their own needs as well as their children's • Having a clear sense of personal values • Valuing independence and autonomy for themselves and their children and acting consistently with these values • Viewing the world with confidence rather than as a dangerous place for themselves and their adolescents • Tolerating experimentation, but having their own limits and therefore being able to keep their own identity intact • Seeing the separation process as a natural part of growth.

Conversely, those parents whom Murphy found to be troubled by separation were parents with a low sense of autonomy and/or of relatedness to other people; parents who were less clear about their own values and identity; and those who were uneasy about communicating differences with others. There was a disparity between their actions and their statements. Closeness and autonomy were problematic for these parents, and they saw the separation process as desertion by their children.

Part II
ADOLESCENT-PARENTAL SEPARATION IN THE CONTEMPORARY MIDDLE-CLASS HOME

CHAPTER 7

The Process of Adolescent- Parental Separation and the Variables Affecting It

Stages of Adolescent-Parental Separation

Although five stages of adolescent-parental separation have been established, it is important to keep in mind that, as with all "stage theories" of human development, the divisions are convenient only for conceptualizing the major issues as one proceeds toward developmental goals. A stage should be reviewed as a heightened sensitivity to learning and development in one area, while development in other areas goes on at a lesser intensity. Movement through these stages is not in one direction but rather, as Bios (1962 pg. 11) points out, "adolescence is a process of regressive and progressive movements appearing and alternating at shorter and longer intervals." This is true for both adolescents and parents in facing the separation process.

The process can be analogized to the steps a skier goes through from the elementary to the advanced level. There are three major techniques, which for consistency will be called stages, that the novice must learn before becoming an advanced skier. These are the snowplow, the stem christie. and the parallel. Each stage has techniques that must be mastered in order to advance. The techniques of the earlier stage must be so integrated that they are largely forgotten while concentrating on the new technique.

Individuals must first learn the snowplow. When this is mastered, they can go down fairly steep hills. Next, they begin to learn the stem christie. Although the technique is somewhat different the edge control of the skis and the balance learned while doing the snowplow are essential to the stem christie. When individuals get into a tough spot, they may automatically return to the snowplow, which is at this stage, more trusted than the new technique. Also, the stem christie is at first not a true technique but a hybrid of snowplow and stem christie techniques. Sometimes, when the skier is feeling quiet confident in a simple situation, a few moments of parallel skiing may be attempted. Little by little, the stem christie is used predominantly and the parallel is tried more frequently. However, even when a considerable degree of confidence has been gained in advanced parallel skiing, if there is a reason for a loss of confidence-an extremely steep mountain, for example-the stem christie or even the snowplow may be relied upon again.

Occasionally, a skier who has not mastered even the elementary snowplow will attempt to parallel ski down a mountain. The result is a fall, sometimes a disastrous one. However, if one proceeds steadily but within the limits of capability, the parallel is eventually mastered and regression to an earlier technique seldom occurs.

Stage 1. The control of the impulse to remain attached. By pubescence, the child is, in many respects, an expert at being a child. The onset of the separation process is often a perplexing experience for both child and parent. Ways of interacting as a child are no longer satisfying to the adolescent. More is open to question. The real cause of the dissatisfaction is often unclear initially, although many explanations may be used to reduce anxiety.

The process of separation begins with an ambivalent push-pull experience by both parents and adolescents. On the one hand, the adolescents desire to test limits, and a greater orientation toward the peer group for these new feelings. Much of this is experienced rather unconsciously, in the form of a desire to be away from home for longer periods, a greater desire to test limits, and a greater orientation toward the peer group for guidance. Furthermore, emerging adolescents begin to question their self-views. It is no longer comfortable to be a child, but neither is it comfortable to be an adult. During this period of time, adolescents often are very concerned about how their parents and others refer to them. In Erikson's terms, identity diffusion has taken place: the childhood identity is being given up.

Adolescents often play down the need for the parents, while at the same time they put themselves in positions of exaggerated dependence. The ambivalence toward the relationship with their parents is sometimes acted out by an exaggerated denial of their need for the parents, while concurrently, then unconsciously force the parents to be parental. For example, a girl I saw in therapy once refused her mother's suggestion to wear a coat on a cold, rainy day. She stayed out in the rain, caught cold, and had to stay in bed, forcing her mother to take care of her.

Parents' response to this is often ambivalent as well as perplexed. They are no longer certain how they should regard their offspring. They are not children, but neither are they adults. The adolescent push-pull is often a confusing message for the parents. The rebellion is often frustrating and angering.

In time, most adolescents and parents recognize this behavior as movement toward independence. Their response at times is to hang on, but eventually most change their orientation to letting go. Their initial stage of separation-the control of impulse to remain attached is successfully resolved, and the second stage begins. This does not mean that the ambivalence toward letting go has been resolved; only the commitment to the ultimate goal has shifted from the maintenance of the attachment to eventual independence.

Stage 2. Cognitive realization of the separation. The main objective of this stage is the cognitive proof and acceptance of separation. Adolescents are very concerned with proving to themselves, as well as to their parents and to the world, that they are indeed separating and becoming more independent. The parents are also involved in gaining a cognitive acceptance of the adolescent's emerging independence.

The initial tentative questioning of limits becomes a continuous bickering between the adolescent and the parents over household rules and limits. In the Offer and Offer (1975) study of Midwestern boys, this was commonplace, and, as they state, "the purpose of the rebellion is to initiate and reinforce emancipation from parents." As the process continues, the disagreements may become broader in subject matter and more abstract, such as arguments over politics, morality, and philosophy of life. By such disagreements, adolescents demonstrate that they have minds of their own. In this context, "different" means "separate" to the adolescent.

Offer and Offer (1975) found that house rules often were broken and other limits tested. The infractions vary, depending on how much limit testing adolescents need in order to prove to themselves and to their parents that they are indeed taking on some of the control previously held by the parents. At times, the cognitive proof of separation will lead adolescents to try alternative styles of dress, philosophical viewpoints, life goals, ego ideals, ethics, morality, and life-styles. This rebelliousness of teenagers is commonly given a negative connotation. Rebelliousness is not necessarily a negative activity, however. Although making parents and other adults often uncomfortable, some rebelliousness aids the separation process.

Some adolescents during this stage develop close interpersonal relationships *only* with people of ethnic or religious backgrounds different from their own. This often occurs when proving differences and separation from parents is particularly difficult, as in the case of a symbiotic relationship.

The differences are often exaggerated by the adolescent when discussing them with parents. Also, parental surrogates, such as teachers, and police, are often rebelled against as a projection of the struggle to prove separation and self-sufficiency. Offer and Offer (1975) found that the boys they studied would often bicker and disagree a great deal at home, while outside of the home many of their allegiances remained true to the most basic values of the parents.

There is a great deal of diversity in the degree and type of rebellion that takes place. What is uniform is that adolescents have to find a way in which to prove to themselves and their parents that they are becoming independent in thought as well as in action (Baittle and Offer 1971). At this point, adolescents are committed only to separation and autonomy. Thus, they are oriented toward rebellion and demonstrating separation. When they have proven to their own satisfaction that they are separate, the rebellion attenuates and the commitment to other goals, philosophies, and so forth becomes possible.

Caught in feeling the need to be less dependent on parental values, yet still uncertain of their own values, adolescents now look more to peers to provide guidelines. As Offer and Offer (1975) point out, although adolescents often find themselves bickering and countering parental limits, there is tremendous uniformity among the peer culture's members. The adolescents are afraid to be outside the limits of their peers. Again, they have no guidelines themselves and therefore are dependent on the peer group for guidelines.

The proof of separation serves as a motivation for attempting more independent functioning as well There is a continual desire for greater spatial and temporal separation from the parent and for greater financial selfsufficiency. This is carried out in activities such as part-time jobs, spending the majority of free time with peers, and going away from home to school. There is, furthermore, an ever-increasing desire to make decisions about the future without parental input.

The parental response to the growing awareness of the adolescent's need for independence is most often a gradual relaxation of parental support and control. This is a difficult time for parents. The continuous testing and rebellion is wearing on them. Because of cultural changes, old guidelines for the rate of allowing more freedom have become less useful. Offer and Offer (1975) found, however, that most of the parents in their sample got used to the continuous bickering and arguing. Those who felt most comfortable with open discussion and argument had the easiest time of it.

By experimenting with different rates of allowing the adolescent more responsibility, parents adjust to the adolescent's changing abilities. As much as adolescents protest parental authority, they derive needed security from it. Parents who too quickly give up control find their adolescent becoming more insecure and forcing more limits by acting out more. Sensitive parents, then, provide more limits, despite protest. Some parents, during this stage, also initiate arguments at times, to show both their caring and their different points of view. Parents who accommodate their views to those of their adolescents in order to avoid conflict only make their adolescents' divergence more extreme, since its purpose is to demonstrate differences. Eventually, adolescents and the parents become more habitually cognizant of their separateness. When this occurs, the third stage begins.

Stage 3. The affective response to the separation. With adolescents and parents accepting the separation on a cognitive basis, the center of focus shifts to the affectual response. Feelings most often described by both parents and adolescents during this stage are those of nostalgia for the past relationship. There is no desire to return to it; in fact, the nostalgia is usually described and felt openly when the separation is most secure. The nostalgia, then, is a feeling response to the acknowledged loss of the child-parent relationship. There is marked variability in how powerfully this nostalgia is felt, ranging from periodic, rambling remembrances of good times spent with the family to deep mourning, despair, and depressive withdrawal. The greater the feelings of mourning and depression during this period, the greater the corresponding feelings of anger and guilt related to the separation. Depression is exacerbated if the anger is denied and/or repressed.

There always appears to be some associated anger and guilt. The guilt is painful to the youth and the response is anger, although this association is often unconscious. The parents often have similar feelings toward the adolescent. When the combination of anger, guilt, and loss combine, periods of depression result, which range from very mild to severe. In this stage, the parents and the adolescent are searching for the meaning of the change in the relationship, for meaning in the death of the childhood identity, and for new goals in a new identity.

For the successful outcome of this stage, guilt and other strong affects must be dealt with successfully. There must also be a basic trust in the relationship, so that an alteration in the direction of greater autonomy would not bring on total rejection and completely destroy the relationship. The adolescent's goal is to be independent, but still to be loved. The parents also want to know that if they accept the adolescent's autonomy, they will still be loved.

Counterbalancing the feelings of loss and associated guilt and anger, happiness and pride are felt by both the parents and the adolescent in seeing the adolescent as an emerging adult. When present, this aids the mitigation process. When the affectual response to the loss has been confronted and, at least to some extent, mitigated, the fourth stage begins.

Stage 4. Identification. At this point, adolescents have faced the feelings associated with separation; they are secure that their identity is now separate from that of their parents, that they are responsible for themselves, and that they have control over making decisions regarding their destiny. Adolescents are then motivated, both consciously and unconsciously, to internalize those qualities of the parents that are of value to them. The adolescent may, in fact, internalize some of the previously rebelled-against qualities, although they may be integrated in a somewhat altered form. For example, the quality of orderliness, which may have been learned in childhood in relation to keeping the house clean, may now be applied to keeping order in one's job, while the house may remain messy. Those traits in parents that are not of value probably will not be reintegrated. Much of what the adolescent sees valuable is a function of what qualities are most valuable to the parents. They may be different, however, from what the parents give lip service to as valuable.

Adolescents must see that parents derive value from a trait or they must feel that a trait is valuable themselves in order to integrate it.

Much of this identification may be unconscious. For example, young women frequently are surprised when they realize that, after rebelling against their mothers for years, they are now, at least in part, parenting their children in a way that is similar to the way in which their mothers parented them.

Although the identification process refers to internalized, valued qualities, the term "value" must be seen in the context of perceived value. In a wider context, an internalized quality may have no value or may even be destructive. For example, a father who smokes is constantly berating himself for it, but it is obvious that he enjoys smoking and, secondarily, enjoys berating himself. Years later his son is smoking and berating himself for maintaining this self-destructive habit. Both father and son are without explanation as to why the son smokes. They say it could not have come from the father-"he is always saying it is dumb to smoke."

As Offer and Offer (1975) and Stierlin (1974) point out, parents must integrate some of the satisfaction derived from their relationship with their children into the process of letting go. For example, a parent who learned to enjoy fishing by taking the children fishing may learn to enjoy fishing with friends or solitarily. This identification process is, however, in healthy developmental separations, quite different from becoming like the adolescent. There are parents, however, who in separating attempt to accommodate to the adolescent's life-style. Very often the results are disastrous. We have all observed and felt sad for the forty-five-year-old mother who attempts to look and act like her twenty-year-old daughter. Our sadness may be caused by unconscious empathy for the mother's ambivalence and pain in letting go of her daughter, that is, her futile attempts to avoid the pain by over-identifying.

The parents' task at this stage is to gain self-esteem from acknowledging that they are successful parents and to internalize the valued aspects of the child-parent relationship and find alternative outlets for it. Through this process the child-parent relationship is given up.

Stage 5. The attenuation of the child-parent relationship and the corresponding development of a new relationship. The final stage is the development of a new relationship between parent and child, based on adultto-adult interaction, and the reintegration of a new identity in both the parent and the emerging adult. For the young adult, this allows for a new openness to intimate relationships with others, the ability to make genuine commitments, and a new sense of stability in identity. Parents may also be developing a new identity, such as mother-in-law or grandparent.

Closeness and distance without guilt between the parent and the young adult can be more comfortably acknowledged, and the closeness can, therefore, be more comfortably acted on by both parties.

The Variables Affecting the Separation Process

The separation process of the adolescent and the parent can occur as tasks that are, at times, challenging and stressful but, overall, as an expected life course leading to personal growth. Under other circumstances, it can be a time of turmoil, which, although painful, can lead to growth and development. It also can lead to self-doubt, a self-imposed restriction of choice, and destructive changes in the life-style.

In their study of adolescent boys in the Midwest, Offer and Offer formulated three developmental routes along which most of their sample families progressed. They refer to these routes as follows: the continuousgrowth group, which comprised approximately 23 percent of the sample; the surgent-growth group, which comprised approximately 35 percent of the sample; and the tumultuous-growth group, which comprised approximately 21 percent of the sample.

Offer and Offer's continuous-growth group came from a "genetically and environmentally excellent background." The main characteristic of this background was stability in the nuclear family, with no serious losses or illnesses of significant others. The environmental and cultural norms were useful and could easily be integrated. Parents were able to adapt to changes as adolescents grew older and to allow for their greater independence. The adolescents had good object relations throughout their development, and the parents projected positive expectations for their children.

In contrast to this, those in the surgent-growth group were more likely to have experienced a traumatic separation, such as a death or illness of a significant person in their life. They developed less self-esteem in their childhood and therefore looked for positive reinforcement from significant others. Some of the mothers had difficulty in letting their children grow up, and there was more conflict between the mothers and the fathers. In the majority of cases, Offer and Offer saw this group as ultimately being as successful in adapting and in their careers and marriages as those of the continuous-growth group. They felt that on the whole, the group was less introspective than either the first or the third group. They felt that the members of the group also were more controlled, with a greater suppression of emotionality than the first group.

The third group, the tumultuous-growth group, was seen as the one most often described in the psychiatric, psychoanalytic, and social science literature. Its members came in contact with the psychiatric community more often than the other groups because of overt behavioral problems, at school or at home, during adolescence. They usually had more conflict in social relations and were inconsistent or did poorly academically. Offer and Offer found that this generally reflected a less stable home environment. The parents more often had overt marital conflict or mental illness. Several in this group were also lower-middle-class teenagers growing up in a middle-class or upper-middle-class environment, which resulted in conflict with the prevailing culture.

This group experienced major psychological trauma. They were not as well equipped to handle emotionally trying situations. Separation was painful to the parents and became a source of continuing conflict for the subjects. Offer and Offer felt, however, that family ties were as strong in this group as in the other two. Once the adolescents had gone through the separation process, they were no less well-adjusted, in terms of their overall functioning, than were the persons in the continuous-growth and surgent-growth group. They usually described themselves more critically and were more critical of their social environment. As a group, they were just as successful academically and vocationally later in life.

In follow-up studies, the continuous-growth group had almost no significant psychiatric syndrome; the surgent-growth group experienced psychiatric syndromes at a rate reflecting the general population; and the tumultuous-growth group had about twice the number of individuals who experienced psychiatric syndromes as the general population. In general, the variables that Offer and Offer see as important to the adolescent- parental separation process are similar to those that will now be discussed. A number of other variables also have an important impact on the separation process.

Variable 1. The readiness of the individual for independence. Is the individual confident in his ability to care for himself? Has he been able to meet life challenges successfully in the past? If he has, the chances are that he will more confidently and comfortably face this life challenge also. More directly, how much experience has he had with independence and taking responsibility? Has he developed confidence from these experiences? In their study, Offer and Offer found that those teenagers who had happy experiences away from home at summer camp or at a part-time job, for example, felt more comfortable facing the separation process.

In close association with experiences of independent functioning, parental expectations of successful, independent functioning are quite influential. For example, has increasing responsibility been placed on the youth for control of impulse? Adolescents who have had more experience with self-regulation can more readily take on responsibility and appear to test out limits of control less than those who have not had as much experience. As a result, they usually face separation with greater confidence and greater selfesteem.

For parents, the issue of "readiness for independence" primarily addresses the confidence they have in finding alternative modes for their generativity and other satisfaction previously derived from their children. These include their sense of purpose, their self-esteem, their creative expression, and, more generally, their exploration of alternatives for interpersonal validation and identity. Do they feel confident in their ability to find alternative outlets for themselves that allow them to feel good about themselves? As Stierlin (1974) points out, those parents who feel they have no alternatives and who are therefore extremely dependent on their children, project these feelings onto their children making the separation process difficult for both. The adolescent usually responds by feeling guilty and angry with the parents' ambivalent behavior.

If the mother and father have good memories of their life together prior to having children, they often feel more confident in their ability to be happy without children. If they were teenage parents, being childless is more of a novelty and more potentially stressful.

Variable 2. Cognitive influences, including object constancy and the assimilative-accommodative modes of adaptation. As described previously, the ability for abstract cognition and the cognitive process of assimilation and accommodation are important variables in the separation process of adolescents. The emergence of formal operational thinking provides the opportunity to reformulate patterns of viewing and experiencing interpersonal relations. The cognitive process is important for rebellion and reinternalization because what is rebelled against and later identified with cannot be separated from what is perceived.

Adolescents who grow up in homes where parents are consistent and where verbalization is an important mode of communication develop the most abstract and complex potential for both rebellion and identification. For those who grow up in homes where there is less verbalization, development in the perception of object relations is more concrete. For example, in a family where verbalization is quite sophisticated, the teenager will more likely discuss subjects such as "making someone feel guilty." As a result, the teenager will understand and recognize the controlling influence of guilt and will likely rebel against the guilt. Teenagers from homes where there is little verbalization regarding guilt would be less likely to recognize its influence and hence not rebel against it. The more complex the ability to formulate patterns of interaction, the greater the awareness (unconscious or conscious) of the parents' subtle influence on the adolescent's behavior.

It follows that adolescents when aware of the parents' subtle influences, will need to rebel against them in order to prove their separateness. Later, they will reidentify with these behavior patterns. Without an awareness of these influences, however, neither rebellion nor identification can take place in response to them. The center of focus for rebellion or identification in the less verbal families may be limited to concrete issues such as leaving the church, whereas, to a more cognitively sophisticated group, issues are often much more subtle and complex, such as styles of child- rearing. The women's movement was formulated and initiated by educated middle-class women, who were able to recognize and formulate the subtle patterns of interaction that are gender related. They recognized the relativity of such patterns, once formulated, to cultural norms rather than seeing them as absolutes. This greater cognitive complexity has the potential for a greater variety and choice of self-definition, both in the direction of more rewarding or more destructive alternatives.

Those who came from homes where parental behavior patterns were inconsistent had the most difficulty in recognizing patterns of relating, as a result, they had problems with rebellion, with identification, and, ultimately, with establishing a self-identity.

With the *development of formal operational thinking* in adolescence, teenagers gain a greater awareness of cultural diversity and become able to compare and evaluate cultural norms. This, in turn, gives adolescents the capability to understand and reevaluate their own norms, values, ethics, and ideals on a higher level of abstraction and complexity. Individuals may use the new abilities to reformulate both their understanding of their relationship with parents and their self-identity. Affecting this reevaluation is the individual's *previous experience in facing novel situations.*

Adolescents may assimilate their observations into their existing childhood frame of reference, may accommodate to an entirely new frame, or may develop an integrated view. Adolescents who in childhood had little education and experience in accommodation will tend to assimilate most of their new experiences into their existing frame of reference. Those who have dealt with novelty by accommodating their views to others' frames of reference will assimilate very' little. Those who have had the opportunity to learn to both assimilate and accommodate novelty will use both cognitive modes in understanding new experiences.

For example, adolescents in our culture are exposed to a diversity of viewpoints on the morality of premarital sex. Adolescents who have had little experience in understanding diversity are likely to be unable to recognize this cultural diversity. They will continue to view morality in their childhood way; that is they will exclusively assimilate their observations of premarital sex into their existing frame of reference. If the parents' view as well as their own childhood view of premarital sex is that it is a sin, they will see it as a sin. They may, in fact, choose to have premarital sex. If they do, it will be seen by them as getting away with a sin.

Adolescents who have had little past experience in successfully understanding diversity but who have a strong need to reject their parents' views are likely to accommodate their views exclusively to those of their peer group. If the peer group believes premarital sex is good, they, too, will believe it.

Adolescents who have had successful experiences in understanding diversity (as explained in Chapter 3) will recognize the diversity of moral viewpoints in our culture. They then have the option of finding a moral view that integrates their assimilative and accommodative cognition. These individuals tend to view morality more relativisticly. They tend to see morality as a pragmatic adjustment to the needs of society and of the individual. They often integrate parental views with those that respond to cultural change.

For parents, cognitive functioning is also an important variable in both object relations and mode of understanding change. The issues of object relations and object constancy are important to them in their being able to separate the needs of the adolescent from their own and to see these needs as sometimes being conflicting. Parents with poor cognition in object constancy regard adolescents as extensions of their own needs; thus, the adolescents' wish to separate is a narcissistic wound. In one family that I saw in therapy, the mother, when she was young, had wanted to be a musician, and she believed that her daughter should also want to be a musician. She could not understand her daughter's questioning of that goal and could not recognize her own needs as distinct from those of her daughter. There is a wide variability of this fusion that parents may have with their children. Indeed, this issue of being able to separate needs exists to a degree in most parents and contributes to the need of youth to rebel. Only in an extreme form does it become pathological. Most parents, through assimilating and accommodating the new reality of their adolescents' growing separateness, come to understand the separation of needs.

The ability to understand novelty through accommodation and assimilation, then, is as important to parents for the separation process as it is to adolescents. Parents who achieved a good integration of assimilation and accommodation were the most successful in facing separation because they were able to see the changes in their adolescents in a context appropriate to the changing world. This allowed them to accurately view and to accept changes in their adolescents, while maintaining the integrity of their own view.

A study of college professors' response to growing student diversity on campuses in the early 1970s illustrates the importance of this cognitive process (Bloom, Ralph, and Freedman 1973). A large sample of faculty was interviewed regarding, among other things, views of changes in students, of student rebellion, and of the importance of authority figures. Some professors were found to have seen students as basically the same as in the past. They felt students were "lazier" because they could get passing grades without being made to work as hard. They saw the goals of students as being the same as when they themselves were students. Student rebellion was seen as a result of the relaxation of strict authority. They felt that students would always act that way in the absence of strict authority. In other words, they assimilated all change into their existing frame of reference.

There were others who, when confronted with diverse views, completely accommodated their views to the students' and who began acting just like students in order to deal with the anxiety aroused by the questions the students posed. They saw only one view or the other as being possible. They accommodated entirely to a new frame of reference.

Another group of professors changed their views of students through an integration of both assimilation and accommodation. They tended to view student change in more relativistic terms. In their view, students were making changes because of changes in the environment in which they were growing up. In this context, these faculty could accept student changes while maintaining what worked well for them (Bloom, Ralph and Freedman 1973).

These general dynamics are equally true for parental views of their adolescents' changes.

Variable 3. The nature of the parent-child relationship. Is it a symbiotic relationship, or is there a mutual respect for independence? How is communication of interpersonal feeling handled? Are overt and covert messages consistent? How are ambivalence, guilt, and anger dealt with? Are parent and child able to discuss feelings and to face them openly? And, most important, is there basic trust, so that both adolescent and parent feel that they can go through a rebellious period where there is anger, ambivalence, and guilt but also basic confidence that there is love and that these feelings will not destroy the relationship?

The separation process is most comfortable when the relationship is secure, yet independence is encouraged. Where dependency has been encouraged, separation is extremely difficult. Where the relationship is symbiotic, separation may be impossible.

> Stierlin (1974), in a study of adolescent runaways, observed a number of parents who though they ostensibly encouraged separation, really communicated that separation was wrong or that it was a rejection of the parents. Stierlin calls this adolescent the "delegate of the parents." Although seemingly free, the adolescent is only free to fulfill the parents' needs. A case in point is the example given previously of the mother who always wanted to

be a musician and who could not understand why her daughter would want to give up music. Giving up her musical career, the mother stated, had been the greatest disappointment of her life. She had given it up to marry and to have a child, her daughter. The underlying message is clear here. The mother would have been a musician if it were not for her daughter. It was, then, the daughter who caused her mother her greatest disappointment, but the daughter could make up for it by becoming a musician for the mother. This, of course, made separation from the mother a nearly impossible task.

The family communication system is also an important aspect of the parent-child relationship. As Bateson (1975), Masterson (1972), Stierlin (1974), and Offer and Offer (1975) point out, where communication is open and congruent, the interpersonal relations are closer and more secure. Double messages, or communication in which the overt and covert messages are disparate, make separation more problematic.

Probably the single most significant feature in determining whether the separation process will be a destructively conflictual one or a developmental one is whether the adolescent feels secure concerning parents' regard for him or her. Since strong affects such as ambivalence, anger, and guilt are always a part of separation, where rejection is seen as likely, separation is seen as dangerous. Furthermore, if the parents are rejecting, then the introjection and identification process includes self-rejection as well.

Another important feature related to the adolescent-parental relationship is how parents exercise authority and control the child's impulse. As Breger (1974) points out, control is at first totally external; as children move away from their parents, they must internalize this control. This learning process may be largely unconscious. As the children grow older, issues of authority and control become more abstract, to include issues of morality and ethics. It is important to the separation process whether the morality is taught by way of shame and punishment or through the use of guilt.

In adolescents' search for cognitive proof of separation, they will use different styles of rebellion and, later, reinternalization as a response to these different approaches. Rebellion against the control taught by shame and punishment usually consists of "getting away with things," or proving that you are now in control of yourself because you can break the rules and get away with it. Thus, one has the choice of following rules or not. However, when control is internalized in the form of guilt, there is no escaping the punishment. In order to rebel against the control, one must change the morality.

Sanford (1970) describes the differences between students attending college during the 1930s, 1940s, and 1950s, when control was maintained largely by external authoritarian methods, and students attending school in the 1960s and 1970s, when control was maintained largely through guilt. The earlier students rebelled by breaking rules such as sneaking out at night, getting drunk, holding panty raids, and the like. This was done largely in the spirit and excitement of rebellion against the control of authority. The authenticity of the authority itself was unquestioned. What is seen more on campuses today, where guilt is largely the method of teaching self-control, is that adolescents will go through a period in which they will change their ethics and moral beliefs, testing out whole new moral systems as a way of rebelling against the control of authority. It is not worthwhile to get away with something if, afterwards, one feels guilty. But, if one changes his or her morality and does something according to the new morality without feeling guilty, one now feels in control.

How ambivalence and anger are dealt with in the adolescent-parental relationship will also have an important impact on the process of separation. Adolescents and parents who are able to deal with these feelings and who regard them as "normal" will have a much easier time than those who have difficulty with ambivalence and anger.

Another important issue is how satisfied the parents feel about their lives, as well as how the adolescent views the parents' feelings of satisfaction. This is important because, if the parental life-style is seen as valuable to the parent, more identification will take place. If it is seen as useless, and if it has not brought satisfaction to the parents, then more of it will be rebelled against and ultimately rejected.

Variable 4. The past experiences of the parents and the adolescent in separation. Offer and Offer (1975) found that those adolescents who experienced a separation from a significant other in childhood were more likely to experience difficulty when separating from their parents. They brought the expectation of the pain from the previous separation to the separation between themselves and their parents.

In contrast, it was found that those teenagers who experienced the separation process most comfortably had had no traumatic separations in their past. Instead, they had separation experiences that correspond to their stage of development-for example, good experiences in going off to nursery school, grammar school, and summer camp, and in outings with high school friends, and so on.

The most important past experience for parents is the experience they had as adolescents separating from their parents. In his study of adolescents and their parents, Stierlin (1974) found that the simultaneous onset of middle age and separation from adolescents encourages parents to review their life and often to reaffirm their loyalty to their own parents and upbringing. He points out that this is to some extent a result of seeing the process of generations and the continuity of life in a larger context. This need to see the continuity of life and generations conflicts somewhat with the adolescent's need to rebel. Whereas the parents are focusing on the continuity among generations, the adolescents are motivated to rebel to find their individuality. This is one reason why it is important for the parents to see the rebellion as part of a process and not as a permanent rejection.

Both Stierlin (1974) and Masterson (1972) point out that those parents who were themselves rejected or who had poor experiences in separating from their parents expected a similar circumstance with their adolescents. To protect themselves from this expected rejection, these parents would often reject their children at the first signs of independence.

The parents' view of their own separation is influenced by other intervening experiences. In reviewing interviews conducted in a longitudinal study of adult life transitions (Lowenthal et al. 1975), Peskin (1977) has observed that the parents' view of separation from their parents is an integration of the remembered reality from adolescence and the reevaluation of it as a result of present circumstances, especially their present relationship with their offspring. That is to say, the existential past of the parents is changed profoundly by their current needs and circumstances.

Variable 5. The cultural influences on the separation process. The present cultural influences on the separation process include the rapid rate of cultural change, the wide cultural diversity, the rapid change of expectation placed on children by adults, and the lack of rituals and guidelines for rites of passage.

The delay and the rapidity of the separation process today compared to past cultures are profound. That is, in modern-day, Western culture, the separation process between parent and adolescent, although initiated psychologically and emotionally at pubescence, actually takes place from eighteen years of age through the early twenties, with little direct preparation such as gradual assumption of adult responsibility. In past cultures, the separation process usually began much earlier and proceeded more slowly, with greater continuity between adolescent and adult responsibilities. Studies of children of nonindustrialized cultures show that they often took care of other children, did chores on the farm, and performed much as they would as adults. Therefore, the transition from childhood to adulthood was much less drastic and much less tumultuous.

The cultural rites of passage, once marked, are now less defined. This has been even more so in the last thirty years than it was before World War II. In the past, the symbols and rituals that usually indicated that the separation process was taking place included the normative passages of men going into the army and being self-supporting and of women getting married and moving out of their home. In the present culture, some of these symbols of separation are still present. However, many eighteen-year-olds go off to college and return home during the summer. This usually means that they are supported, at least in part, by their parents, and therefore separation and independence are much less clearly defined than in the past. As a result, parents and adolescents do not agree on when separation has taken place. In a study in which eighteen-year-olds and their parents were asked if the adolescent was independent, the majority of the youths answered that they were, while the majority of the parents answered that they were not (Peskin 1977). Therefore, there is often a much greater need for the young adult to define and to prove separation, that is, more rebellion.

In past cultures, mentor relationships were built into the cultural system. A mentor can be extremely valuable in the adolescent's emergence into adulthood; unfortunately, the opportunity to have a mentor today is subject to chance, and many have no mentor relationship. As Levinson et al. (1970) points out, even those who do have a mentor find one rather late, that is, as they enter a professional career some years past adolescence.

Another important aspect of the culture is how rapidly it is changing. In order to be successful in the midst of this rapid change, adolescents must strongly question their parents' ways of doing things. They must consider whether their ways are still relevant and successful in the present environment.

The greater choice in today's culture means more questioning of cultural norms. In Europe during medieval times, there was only one right and one wrong; no one thought about whether to accept the cultural norms. After the New World colonies had been established, people became aware of alternate cultural norms. It was possible then for them to question Old World norms, to feel as though they had a choice. Contemporary culture appears to offer unprecedented diversity and choice. Teenagers' fluid identity, combined with wide cultural diversity, make them look more to the peer group for a set of norms and support. Good peer relations are therefore extremely important to the adolescent during the process of separating from parents.

If, at some point, the rate of change slows and the culture becomes less diverse, we may find that when today's adolescents become parents, they may expect to face more rebellion than what will occur. They may be as perplexed with the lack of rebellion as many parents from less rebellious backgrounds today are perplexed at their offspring's rebelliousness. Peskin (1977) points out that this dynamic is, in fact, occurring in the Israeli kibbutzim.

In summary, today's culture puts greater stress on the parents and the adolescents than in previous times. This makes the parent-child relationship even more significant today to a successful outcome of separation than it has been in the past.

CHAPTER 8

Case History of Wayne Marlie

Introduction

Wayne Marlie's[2] separation from his parents is representative of the experiences of middle-class teenagers and parents today. As with most middle-class parents and adolescents, they faced the separation experience with little understanding of what they were going through. For Wayne and his parents the experience was stressful at times, but it is one which has been resolved productively, with family members having gained from the experience. The case, then, demonstrates how these people faced and resolved the issues of the separation process with little direct understanding of its dynamics.

Wayne Marlie was interviewed in the context of a study of the psychosocial development of college students. The interviews particularly stressed how the students' past and their being away from home for the first time affected their personal development.

Wayne was chosen from a large number of possibilities because, over a two-year period, his history became more completely documented than many others who were interviewed. He was open and lucid in the interviews, as well as in less formal conversations. He enjoyed the interviews and was interested in the study and therefore enthusiastically gave as much information as time allowed. As a result, it was possible to gather much more information about him than about others in the sample.

Wayne was interviewed at approximately three-month intervals during his freshman and sophomore years. He was eighteen when the interviews began and nearly twenty at their completion. The interviews covered material related to his background and past, including the significant events of his childhood. The interviews focused especially on his relationship with his parents and on how it changed during the period of the study.

The information in the case history has been drawn from Wayne's account. Therefore, it cannot be considered entirely objective. Pains were taken to separate information that was obviously subjective interpretation from that which appeared objective. The material in this case must be considered as being filtered through Wayne's experience, but as this case is a demonstration rather than a proof of the thesis of this book, this fact should not take away from its value. As with clinical case studies, changes in Wayne's perceptions may be used as further data as well.

Wayne was a white male of medium height and build, and he appeared good-looking. During interviews he was usually dressed in blue jeans, a sport shirt, and tennis shoes, all of which appeared clean. During the last year of our interviews, he wore a mustache and allowed his hair to grow to almost shoulder length.

The Childhood Environment

Both of Wayne's parents were white, Anglo-Saxon protestants. Around the time of his birth, the family was considered middle class. Mr. Marlie was a carpenter who went into business for himself as a contractor not long after Wayne's birth. This caused the family to be financially strapped for several years. However, Mr. Marlie eventually became more successful, and in five or six years the family began living at a level that would be considered upper middle class. They had little financial difficulty during this period, except for short times when the building industry became depressed. These usually lasted only a year or so, and, while it put financial pressure on the family, it did not change their life-style dramatically.

The family lived, and still lives, in a suburban area of a large metropolitan city on the West Coast. They moved only once, when Wayne was about five years old, into a fairly large house in what was then a semirural area, but which quickly became suburbanized.

For the most part, the area is politically conservative, as were Mr. and

Mrs. Marlie. The family attended church irregularly, mainly for special occasions such as Easter, although the Marlie children attended Sunday school for a number of years when they were young. Church was seen more as a duty or tradition than as an integrated part of family life. The Marlie children attended well-budgeted public schools in the area.

Wayne's Mother

Mrs. Marlie was born in 1925 to a lower-middle-class family. She grew up in Los Angeles during the Depression; although money was always a problem, her family was never desperate financially.

Mrs. Marlie had a close relationship with her parents. In general, the family was close-knit. There were no real issues of discipline between the parents and the children. Everybody knew what was expected of him or her and did it without much discussion. Mrs. Marlie was considered a good child. She respected and looked up to her parents. The family was rather religious, attending church regularly, and the Christian faith was considered an important part of their daily life.

Mrs. Marlie's goals in life were traditional for the time. She wanted to get married, raise a family, and attain financial security. She talked to Wayne of feeling stifled in adolescence and of not being able to do a lot, blaming it on the Depression and the lack of money rather than on parental control. She met Mr. Marlie while they were both in high school. He was a senior at the time, and she was a freshman. He went into the service soon afterwards, and she saw him only when he was on leave. She dated other men during this time.

When she was a senior in high school they became engaged, and soon after her graduation in 1943 they were married. Her parents felt that she should not marry so young, but they consented. Ambivalent feelings about leaving home may have existed but were very subtly expressed. For example, during the engagement her parents often asked if she was sure of her plans. After her marriage she worked as a secretary near her parents' home. Following the war, Mrs. Marlie worked for a couple more years as a secretary and then became pregnant with Wayne. The pregnancy was untroubled, and Mrs. Marlie was a proud, happy mother. The financial situation of the family during this period was precarious. However, Mr. Marlie became more successful in his business and, as time went on, the financial woes of the family were alleviated. They bought a new house. Mrs. Marlie became pregnant two years after Wayne was born. These were happy years for Mrs. Marlie. She was a proud mother, she had financial security, and she generally felt satisfied with life.

She related to Wayne that she looked to Dr. Spock, as well as to her own mother, for advice in raising her children. She felt confident in her abilities as a mother. This satisfaction with life generally continued unchanged until Wayne reached pubescence, when a rather difficult period for Mrs. Marlie began. She was filled with some doubt and uncertainty about her own future and questioned herself about her abilities. This will be discussed in more detail when Wayne's adolescence is discussed.

Mrs. Marlie was very outgoing, considered pleasant to be with, and had many friends. Within the family, she was able to show her feelings of pleasure, concern, and sadness openly. She was less comfortable with expressing her anger. When she was angry she became temporarily withdrawn, pouted, and showed a general feeling of disappointment, but not in words.

In general, Mrs. Marlie was satisfied with her life and had a generally optimistic view of life. She experienced mild, normal ups and downs; had good defenses of denial and sublimation; and evidently had some histrionic modes to deal with unpleasant feelings. For example, she would sometimes deal excitedly with an issue in avoidance of a more troublesome issue.

Wayne's Father

Mr. Marlie was born in 1923. He was from a lower-middle-class area of Los Angeles. Mr. Marlie's mother and father were not particularly close with each other, at least not overtly. However, they got along reasonably well, respected each other, and were generally secure in their relationship. Mr. Marlie loved and respected both his parents. He felt that they tried to be good parents and were always concerned about him.

The family was not particularly religious and rarely, if ever, attended church. The father was the disciplinarian. Mr. Marlie felt that discipline from his father was rather abrupt but just. Mr. Marlie was not a major discipline problem as a child, although he did get into occasional squabbles with his siblings.

Mr. Marlie grew up in the Depression as well, and his family was continually troubled by financial burdens. As a result, Mr. Marlie worked during much of his high school career at part-time jobs. He was an average student, doing well enough to get by and to graduate. During adolescence Mr. Marlie sometimes got into trouble for pranks, for being home late, for missing school, and for other such limit testing. He got into a few arguments with his father over rules but expressed most of his rebellion to peers in rap sessions. Following his graduation, he joined the military service, as the war in Europe was going on and the United States was expected to enter it shortly. He was dating Mrs. Marlie at that time. He became engaged to her in 1942, and they were married in 1943. Because of his family's financial uncertainty during the Depression years, he was determined that his children would have financial security and a comfortable life. Following the war, he apprenticed as a carpenter. After several years learning the trade, he decided to go into business for himself and began a contracting firm. Mr. Marlie had been an extremely hard worker his whole life, took a lot of pride in his work, and often worked longer than forty hours a week. Such dedication and aggressiveness in his work paid off in his success in the contracting business.

Mr. Marlie took great pride in providing a secure, financially healthy environment for his family, and it is this contribution that he gave as a demonstration of his caring for them.

Mr. Marlie related to Wayne that, when Wayne was born, he felt proud to be a father. However, he spent little time with his first child until the child was older. He left most of the caring of the children before the age of three or four to their mother. When Wayne was three or four, and his younger sister, Lori, had been born, Mr. Marlie began to take a growing interest in his son. He began to play with him and felt more comfortable in their interaction. He became increasingly interested as Wayne became older and participated in many activities with him such as athletics and camping trips. He became involved with the Cub Scouts and, later, the Boy Scouts, when Wayne joined. When his daughter became older, he took more interest in her as well, playing and interacting with her much more. However, he had much less interaction with Lori than with Wayne, primarily because she was not involved with athletics. He felt that she should be feminine and spend more time with her mother. He always supported his daughter when she did something well—for example, in school.

Mr. Marlie was the ultimate disciplinarian for the children. When Mrs. Marlie felt that the children were not responding to her, the threat was to tell Mr. Marlie when he came home. When Mr. Marlie came home, he followed through as the supplier of discipline. This usually consisted of yelling at the children, which seemed to have more impact than the mother's yelling at them, since she did it more frequently. His demonstrations of caring, on the other hand, were often nonphysical, such as giving presents, offering advice, and other indirect expressions of affection. It appears that both children were very secure in regard to his affection for them.

Mr. Marlie was described by Wayne as an easy-going, politically conservative man, who was somewhat shy and quiet around strangers but outgoing and with a good sense of humor around his friends. His son described him as being somewhat bigoted in his jokes, although in direct contact with people he was, evidently, a fair man with almost everyone. Some of the people who worked for him were minority people, and he treated everyone equally. He often enjoyed such activities as drinking beer with his buddies and talking sports. He was able, in the family, to show anger and disapproval openly. He had more difficulty showing his feelings of weakness and his dependency on his wife. He was the acknowledged leader in the family, although decisions were much more mutual than was openly admitted. That is, his wife had a lot more control in the family than either of them openly acknowledged.

He had strong defenses against uncomfortable feelings, such as feelings of insecurity. He dealt with these feelings in an obsessive-compulsive style-for example, developing household rules to deal with uncomfortable feelings in the family.

Wayne's Sister

Lori is almost three years younger than Wayne. Wayne always felt very close to Lori. As a youngster, he was very protective of her, and she looked up to him and enjoyed that protection. Wayne felt that he and Lori received equal love from both parents, although they were, in some respects, treated differently. Less pressure for academic success was placed on Lori than on her older brother. Lori was a good student, although satisfied with less than excellence, which was in contrast to her brother. She was very socially oriented, had lots of girl friends and usually had a boy friend. She was seen by her parents as a "good" girl. The siblings often got into squabbles, but on the whole they got along well. Lori felt very close to both her mother and father.

At pubescence, Lori began getting into many more squabbles with both her mother and her father, usually with regard to limits of control, such as curfews. Lori believed that she should get more freedom than she was granted. Her father often let it be known that the boy Lori was interested in at the time was not good enough for her. He obviously did not want to let go. At the time of the interviews with Wayne, Lori was in her junior year of high school, and over the course of the interviewing she became a senior. She was a better-than-average student and had a steady boyfriend. The arguments between Lori and her parents became more frequent during the course of the interviews. It appears that guilt, confusion, and self-doubt were experienced by both Lori and her parents. She was also doing some limit testing, such as coming in late, but generally stayed within the expectations of her parents.

Family Dynamics

The family was very child-centered, especially when the children were younger. The orientation was "What was good for the children was good for the family." The children's welfare always came first.

Between the parents, there were rarely outward displays of affection, but both obviously derived a general feeling of security and a sense of selfworth from the relationship. There appeared to be genuine closeness between the parents.

The recognized leader of the family was Mr. Marlie. Mrs. Marlie outwardly demonstrated her dependency on him. When major decisions were to be made, however, it was obvious that there was greater mutuality of input, as previously stated. When Mrs. Marlie disagreed with her husband's decision, she would indirectly show her disapproval-for example, by pouting and encouraging guilt in her spouse-and thus gain considerable influence. On the whole, Mr. and Mrs. Marlie seemed generally to agree on most issues.

When the children were young, the family spent a lot of time together, taking camping trips and so forth. Family members generally enjoyed time together and looked forward to special occasions, such as family picnics, going to the beach, holiday celebrations, family gatherings, and going to visit relatives.

There was a great deal of verbal communication within this family. Even nonverbal messages such as pouting were verbalized by other members of the family for example, Wayne's father yelling at his wife, "Your pouting isn't going to make me change my mind," thus verbalizing guilt and control associated with pouting behavior.

During adolescence, both Lori and Wayne were less eager to go on family outings and wanted more freedom to pursue their own interests. During major family events, for example, at Christmas, the family still looked forward to being together, but on weekends and lesser holidays, the adolescents more and more wanted to do things on their own.

Wayne's Developmental History

Mrs. Marlie's pregnancy and Wayne's birth were uncomplicated. He was a healthy baby and was breast fed for several months. Developmental milestones were within normal limits. He was, as stated previously, well loved by both parents, although his father left the responsibility for his early care to Mrs. Marlie. For issues such as toilet training, Mrs. Marlie primarily looked to Dr. Spock, her mother, the general cultural norms, and her peer group for guidelines.

When Wayne was four years old, his parents sent him to nursery school for several hours a day. They felt that it would be good preparation for his attending kindergarten the next year.

When Wayne started school, he was an excellent student and got good grades, usually among the best in his class. He received strong support and encouragement from home for excelling in school. Wayne states that when he brought home his A's, his father would "strut around like a peacock with a smile."

As his father showed more interest in him, Wayne became interested in athletics and outdoor activities. He became a member of the Cub Scouts and excelled in the activities.

He was considered a good boy, although at times he got into some mischief with his friends such as in sneaking off the school yard during lunchtime or in undertaking a Halloween prank. His parents punished him for these transgressions, although they felt that these represented normal growing-up kinds of behavior.

When Wayne did get into trouble, he usually received punishment, such as being yelled at. For more severe transgressions, he might get sent to his room for a period of time or possibly be spanked. He was rarely spanked when very young and not at all by age ten. Usually a spanking was more distressing in its embarrassment and shame than its physical pain, as he really was not hit hard. Wayne stated that the discipline that had the most impact on him was when his parents showed their disappointment in him. The guilt he felt as a result of disappointing his parents was quite painful to him. His parents were aware of this and evoked this response rarely and only in response to issues they saw as very serious—for example, when he shoplifted a toy.

The first times that Wayne could remember being away from home was spending days with his grandmother. This was a regular occurrence, which he remembers as enjoyable. At the age of eight, he spent a weekend at a Cub Scout camp and had positive memories of that experience. As he grew older, he went on much longer excursions with the Cub Scouts and then went away from home during the summer to Boy Scout camp. He remembered this favorably.

The first time he experienced a painful separation was at the age of ten when the family cat died. He remembered crying over its loss. He also remembered having bad dreams for a time afterwards. He had no memory of how he got over those feelings; they just ended on their own. Another separation Wayne remembers as significant was his best friend's moving away when he was fifteen. He had no best friend for about six months following that, although he had casual friends. These feelings also attenuated after a time. He remembered his parents as very supportive after each of these losses.

In his childhood, he viewed his father as being the "strong one," the security in the family, the smart parent, and a fair judge. He felt proud of and very close to his father and looked up to him. He saw his mother as the weaker of the two, more vulnerable in her feelings toward him, and more sensitive and dependent on the father. She was a great source of security for him; she was there when he was hurt, when he needed a sympathetic ear, and when he needed warmth and nurturing. Just as with his father, he was very proud of his mother and felt very close to her.

At the time of pubescence, a number of important changes began occurring in Wayne's relationship with his parents. Wayne's perception of his mother began changing. He began to see her as more and more overprotective, trying to direct him when he felt he did not need direction. He also became more critical of his father. His father fell off his pedestal during this period. Wayne no longer saw him as perfect and no longer wanted to be just like him. In fact, he was angered by every new disillusionment; he felt as though he had somehow been duped. His father, as Wayne later realized, had in no way tried to present himself as irreproachable. He remembers his father saying, "Before, I was perfect; now I can't do anything right."

Wayne had seen his father as a hero because of his own needs for attachment; now, as he needed to separate, his father became a fallen idol. Since one is always aware of one's own flaws, he must see others as flawed before he can regard himself as their equal. It was probably the beginning of a desire to see himself as an equal that made Wayne bring his father down from hero-worship.

Wayne and his parents began to get into frequent arguments. After some of these arguments Wayne felt guilty, although he never expressed this to his parents. His guilt likely contributed to greater anger. The major outlet for his feelings was frequent bickering over what the rules and limits for him should be and what right the parents had to make the rules.

At times he would test out rules—for example, by coming in late. He and his parents would often have long discussions, arguments, half-discussions and half-arguments with him. His parents appeared uncertain as to how much freedom Wayne should be allowed. They slowly gave more freedom to him, and, if he handled it well, they gave him a little more, such as later curfews and a driver's license. It never appeared to be fast enough for Wayne. At times Mr. and Mrs. Marlie felt hurt by Wayne's rejection and rebellion. In the initial interviews, Wayne responded to his parents' hurt with anger. He complained, "They lay these trips on me and then they are hurt; it's bullshit!" In the last of the interviews, Wayne was more open to the pain that his parents felt during this period, as well as to his own guilt in response to it. He related, "It bothered me to see my parents so troubled by my actions, but I had to break free."

Without his parents to rely on for direction, Wayne looked more and more to his peers. He had a number of friends and, except for one brief period, always had a best friend. On the whole, this peer group came from friends who shared similar backgrounds. They, too, were middle class and close to their parents but were going through the same sorts of battles over freedom and control. The peer group put pressure on its members to be independent. The more independence one could get from one's parents, the higher the status in the group. This increased as Wayne grew older. For example, he felt very embarrassed when, at fifteen, he was out on a date and his mother picked up him and his date from the theater.

During high school, athletics were important to Wayne, and he was on several teams. He received letters, but was not an outstanding athlete.

At fifteen, as noted previously, Wayne was without a best friend. He had friends, but he was more alone during this time. He did not remember this as a particularly depressed time; he just felt like being alone. After about six months, he had another best friend.

During his senior year in high school, much of the same interaction with his parents continued, although the bickering became less pronounced and much of the discussion turned to more philosophical and moral disagreements. His parents allowed him more freedom, such as camping trips with his friends, as he became older. During some of these trips, his friends sneaked some liquor, and he got drunk a few times. He tried marijuana once during his senior year. Also during his senior year, he persuaded his parents to allow him to buy a car with the money he had made from his summer job at a hamburger stand. For him the car was a symbol of independence, and among his friends it was a symbol of prestige.

During Wayne's sophomore year in high school, he and his parents had decided that it would be a good idea for him to go away to college, and during his senior year, he took the necessary tests and applied to a number of schools, all away from home. He finally settled on a small liberal arts university about fifty miles from his home, which had an experimental college concentrating on an integration of academics with social action. When he went off to college some major changes occurred, both in his relationship with his parents and in his self-identity.

Wayne lived in the dormitory the first part of his freshman year, and then he moved out and lived with two male roommates for the rest of the year. He was not very interested in school at this point, but he engaged in a lot of self-education such as reading, especially in philosophy. He was, at times, argumentative with his teachers in a competitive way.

He was active outside school, spending a lot of time traveling with his friends. He became mildly involved with drugs, primarily smoking marijuana on the weekends. He once took LSD to find out about himself and stated that it was an interesting experience but one that he did not plan to repeat because he failed to find out much about himself.

During that first year he was also pressured by the Selective Service and had a lot of difficulty deciding what he would do if he were drafted. He considered being a conscientious objector, going to Canada, or just allowing himself to be drafted. To his great relief, he was eventually excused from the service because of his high lottery number.

In the latter part of his first year of college, Wayne thought of taking time off to work. Just before school let out, he got a job but decided to return to school the next year.

Wayne made several new, good friends during that first year. He kept in touch with two of his old high school friends, but he was shifting his peer group orientation to his college friends. He also became politically active in his first year at college. This was during the Vietnam War era, and he participated in some protests. He was opposed to any kind of violence. At the same time, he thought it was very important to make his belief in the peace movement heard.

During his freshman year, Wayne sought peer support as he and close friends investigated and shared ideas on alternative politics, life-styles, and morality; many of these attitudes were in contrast to his parents' beliefs. He grew his hair long and wore clothes that were associated with the contemporary hippy movement. He was uncommitted to any definite lifestyle and was primarily interested in exploring and experimenting; he felt that he had the freedom to experiment.

His questions regarding morality had limits and were often idealized forms of his parents' morality, even though he talked about them rebelliously. Those issues of morality that seemed to be universally held by all cultures, such as not stealing and nonviolence, he professed in their most idealized forms.

Wayne's pluralistic cultural environment was one in which he observed many alternative life-styles. He came into contact with alternative views on sexual morality, dress standards, religion, what obligations the society has to the individual, and whether one owes the society a military career. These were all things that he questioned although he went through periods of believing different things. Most important, he became conscious of the relativity of the answers; that is, what was right at one time may not have been at another time.

He went out with a number of young women and had sexual relations with one he liked. He did not feel committed to any of them. At times he expressed concern that he could not love because he had not fallen in love with any of these young women.

Wayne's relationship with his parents changed considerably during this period. The issue of limits was less important following his departure from home. He usually returned home for a visit about one weekend every two months. During these visits the focus of their discussions was their differences in philosophies of life and morality. At that point, Wayne was very critical of his parents' inconsistencies. Usually when he went home there was little conflict the first day and they would have a good time, but by the second day they would get into an argument, usually about philosophical issues.

During this period Wayne also became critical of the entire peer group to which his parents belonged. The white Anglo-Saxon upper-middle-class culture became a focus for his criticism. He changed philosophies frequently. On different occasions he believed in humanistic psychology, Zen Buddhism, and social conflict theory. At first he would be excited about a belief system, but eventually he would become disenchanted with it and would move on to another one. His parents often responded to this by feeling upset and rejected, and then did not understand how Wayne could change this way. At times they feared for their child and felt angry at the rejection. Basically, however, they had confidence in Wayne's being a good person and felt that he would ultimately find what would be a valuable philosophy for him to live by. They further believed that, in the really important issues of morality, he had high character.

Wayne's parents continued to support his increased self-responsibility. During his second year of college, instead of paying for his individual expenses, they put him on a budget. They would give him a lump sum at the beginning of each semester, and he was responsible for making that money last the entire time. The amount of money was figured out by Wayne and his parents together. He always asked for a lower sum than his parents finally gave him. He felt some guilt about rejecting their philosophies on the one hand and accepting the rewards of their life-style on the other. The summer after his first year, Wayne got a job with the forest service, clearing firetrails. He worked very hard, really enjoyed it, and felt very good about earning a decent salary. He saved a good portion of the money for his schooling, but it only reduced his parents' contribution by about one-fourth.

When Wayne returned to school, he moved into a house with two males and two females. After three months he decided that he wanted to live by himself and moved into his own apartment. In his second year he became somewhat disenchanted with left-wing politics in particular and other politics in general. He also lost interest in philosophical pursuits. He became more interested in school, and during his second year his grades improved markedly.

At the same time, he became less critical of his parents and got along better with them. They were more accepting of his beliefs, and he was more accepting of theirs. What he had previously heard from his father as orders now sounded more like advice. He felt free to either accept or reject it. He still felt guilt and anger at times, but he got over it more quickly and could see their differences in greater perspective. When he visited his parents, he felt that he was treated on a more equal basis.

When Wayne left home on one occasion, he felt depressed. What stuck out in his mind on this visit was the fact that his bedroom had been changed around to make it more of a guest room. He was treated as a loved guest in his parents' home, in other words, more as an equal. He said that for the first time, he felt that he was really alone in the world. He felt sad and fearful. At the same time, he felt a real pride in the feeling of being more on his own.

Following this visit, he reminisced frequently about times that he had spent with his parents when he was younger, and, for the first time, he felt like those times were really over. He felt closer to his parents than he had in years. He also noticed that his parents were beginning to enjoy their independence from him. This relieved him. He stated that his parents were planning a trip to Mexico in a camper they had recently bought. Furthermore, his mother was looking for work. To Wayne it symbolized the fact that his parents were beginning to get involved in some new things that did not include him but that were enjoyable to them. He did not have to feel guilty anymore for not being part of the family; they could enjoy life without him.

They still got into occasional arguments, but he felt much less critical of them. He could see their points of view in the context of their upbringing and environment. Although he sometimes argued, he did not feel that the disagreements were very important anymore.

During his sophomore year some important social changes also occurred. He was falling in love with a girl he had known from the previous year; he now felt much closer to her and saw her in a new way. They considered living together the next year.

In describing himself, Wayne stated that over the past year he had become less idealistic and more skeptical toward politics and that there really was no utopia. He also recognized that he actually believed some of his parents' ideas that he had rejected. For example, he wanted to be successful in a traditional career. He was much more interested in school, and he was doing quite well. He was especially interested in anthropology and law and felt that he would probably go into one of those two fields. He was actually trying to figure out a way in which to integrate those two interests into some specialty, such as studying the roots of law or international law. He did not know how to do it at this point, but he was looking for a creative integration.

In the interviews during the second year, Wayne was increasingly selfconfident, casual, and comfortable, and was less deferent. In general, he seemed to regarded himself as closer to being the equal of the interviewer, a reflection of his change in self-view.

CHAPTER 9

Discussion of Wayne Marlie's Separation from His Parents

Wayne's separation process included struggle and pain, both for himself and for his parents. However, they were all able to meet the challenges well, and, as a result, the experience not only led to a more mature independence for Wayne but also enabled both Wayne and his parents to learn a great deal from each other. Wayne's separation will be discussed first in terms of the stages of separation that were presented in Chapter 1 and will be followed by a discussion of the variables involved in this process.

The Stages in Wayne's Separation

Stage 1. Control of impulse to reattach. The beginnings of Wayne's separation process were not clearly defined. At the age of about twelve to fourteen, he began to see his mother as overprotective, and he wanted to do things more independently. At the same time, he became critical of his parents. A mood of perplexing dissatisfaction was a hint that he had begun to feel ambivalent about his dependence on his parents. Previously he saw his father as a perfect model, someone whom he would want to follow and imitate. These two coincidental changes in attitude toward his parents were probably the beginnings of the separation process, and they reflected the first confrontation with his *impulse to remain attached.* Initially, these feelings led to intermittent arguments with his parents. After a while the arguments became more frequent, and anger was associated with this critical attitude toward his parents. At this point both Wayne and his parents were perplexed by their arguments. The child-parent relationship had been going well, and Wayne had been considered a good child. All of a sudden the parents had fallen off the pedestal; he was angry at them, and they were angry and hurt by this change.

There was also identity diffusion. Wayne no longer wanted to be regarded as a child. His parents were unsure as to how much freedom to give him and how to respond to his anger. Whereas it was very clear to them before as to how much responsibility should be given to Wayne, it was now less clear. At this point, both parents and Wayne were ambivalent about letting go.

As time passed, Wayne and his parents became increasingly aware that independence was the issue and began to accept the eventual outcome, although what "independence" meant was as yet unclear. The arguments between Wayne and his parents continued, but now seen in the proper context, they were recognized as part of a process and were less perplexing. With the shift in emphasis from maintaining the attachment to that of separation, the first stage concluded.

Stage 2. The cognitive realization of the separation. The second stage of the separation process was reflected in Wayne's rebellion against parental limits and influence. How much responsibility Wayne should be given was subject to argument. Furthermore, Wayne began to argue with his parents over philosophies of life. He experimented with dress styles and became committed to philosophical utopias, the nature of which he changed frequently. All of these things were in opposition to his parents' beliefs. The parents' morality and view of reality was questioned. Wayne was working hard at being different from his parents, at discovering and proving to himself and to his parents that he was in fact different. He-focused on the differences, because being different at this point meant not being under the influence of his parents, that is, being independent of them.

Wayne also took on more self-responsibility. First, he bought a car, which, to American youth, was a symbol of freedom and independence, or adulthood. Second, he decided to go away to college, and his parents supported his decision. He was excited but apprehensive about the decision, as were his parents.

When Wayne got to college he began to try out alternative living styles and philosophies of life. An example was his moving into the coeducational house. In this environment he attempted to find a utopian living situation and also searched for utopian politics. He also began to feel ambivalence toward accepting money from his parents. He gained some financial independence by getting a part-time job.

The parents' responded to this rebelliousness with sadness and anger; they felt rejected. However, they recognized that this rebellion was part of the separation process. They encouraged Wayne to take more responsibility as they slowly relaxed their control over limits. Although it was difficult for them, they recognized and acknowledged Wayne's increasing ability to function independently. However, they still felt that rejection of their belief system was a rejection of their parenting. Still, they were able to trust the basic soundness of Wayne's character. This trust asserted their basic love for Wayne and their basic confidence in their own judgment. At times they made Wayne feel guilty for his behavior, but more often they discussed their disagreements openly. Along with supporting Wayne's widening breadth of responsibility, they began thinking about and planning for more independence for themselves. As time went on, Wayne and his parents became more aware of his ability to take care of himself and to make life choices for himself.

Stage 3. The affective response to the separation. As Wayne entered his second year of college, he and his parents argued less frequently; they accepted their independence and their differences on a cognitive level. At that point Wayne expressed to the interviewer feelings of guilt resulting from the arguments. Later he wondered, "Why did I argue?" This greater awareness of his guilt appeared to reflect a more pervasive openness to his parents' sadness at separating from him. At that time, when the arguments were on the wane and the separation was closer to resolution, there was actually less to feel guilty about. It was then that Wayne was more conscious of his guilt feelings. Most likely, the attenuation of the guilt in the relationship allowed him to be more open to it.

At that time, Wayne felt a sense of his aloneness in the world. The arguments with his parents reminded him of that aloneness, and he felt sad. He went home for a visit at that point and found that his room was set up more as a guest room than as "his room." While at home, he was treated more as a guest and more equally. He responded to the change with pangs of nostalgia. During that visit he and his parents reminisced about what it was like when he was a child. After he returned to school, he periodically reflected on the change in his room and felt more pangs of nostalgia. Now that the separation was more secure, he could consciously feel the sadness associated with it. He began to develop a more skeptical attitude toward utopian ideas, which reflected a movement toward not focusing so completely on the differences between himself and his family.

His parents also showed more nostalgia when he left from his visits. Whereas previously they had often gotten into arguments with him as he was leaving, they now expressed sadness about his going back to school. They were also more open to their own feelings of nostalgia and sadness in the separation. However, Wayne, and his parents felt a pride in his growing independence. His parents talked about how he was really becoming a man, and Wayne was feeling like a man. The guilt associated with the separation was also becoming more open; for example, Wayne felt a certain fear and guilt that his parents could not enjoy themselves without their children. When they used to go on camping trips together, the children were very much a part of their fun. The parents, however, were reassuring as they made plans for trips on their own. Some of Wayne's fears may have been a projection of his own sadness and his inability to enjoy freedom as much as he wanted to. During Wayne's second year in college, along with the nostalgia and guilt he expressed anger in response to these feelings for his parents. As time passed, these feelings were mitigated more and more.

Stage 4. Identification. Wayne began to recognize similarities that he had with his parents toward the end of his second year at college. At first he was ambivalent about this recognition, since it implied ambivalence toward accepting his own inadequacies. As he became more able to provide for himself, his own guidelines became more comfortable, his need for utopian goals diminished, and he began to commit himself to more realistic goals. This included reaccepting values that he had learned from his parents. He desired a career in anthropology or law, which was very much in keeping with the values of his parents. This ability to accept himself and others more realistically, as well as his growing acceptance of his emerging adult identity, gave him the freedom to be more involved in heterosexual relationships. He became increasingly close to a woman. In this relationship he recognized further his identification with his parents. For example, the importance he placed on monogamy, a value he had in common with his parents, became clear to him. Prior to this awareness, he focused so much on how he and his parents differed that he did not recognize the similarities. This is not to say that he did not retain some of his individual differences. He wanted his career in law or anthropology to be somewhat nontraditional; for example, he wanted to integrate law and anthropology in a creative way that would be an expression of himself. This was an integration of Wayne's experience and goals with those that came from his developmental background with his parents. This integration came about as a result of activities oriented toward finding his individuality and, once it was found, toward reaccepting the influence of his parents.

With the struggle for separation more resolved, Mr. and Mrs. Marlie were redefining themselves as parents with grown children. Their acceptance of their own independence was shown, for example, in their desire to enjoy by themselves activities that they once shared with their children. They planned a trip on their own and bought a camper for themselves. They became committed to enjoying life in a new way, with each other and without the children. This gave Wayne "permission" to feel more comfortable in separating. The purchase of a camper may have been further encouraged by an identification on the parents' part of the new freedom of their children, which they saw as desirable for themselves as well.

Stage 5. The attenuation of the child-parent relationship and the corresponding development of a new relationship. Although the separation process was not complete at the time the interviews ended, there was evidence of the beginning of the final stage. Both Wayne and his parents began to see themselves as more equal in the relationship.

Wayne felt an identity separate from his parents. He felt comfortable making future plans on his own. He saw his parents more realistically as products of their environment and could accept them as important people who were different and separate from himself. He could accept faults in his parents as well as be critical of himself. When his parents gave him advice, he could hear it as advice and not as commands or as his parents talking down to him. However, there were still times when he and his parents regressed for short periods to earlier ways of interacting. It was obvious, however, that the process would be completed with both the parents and Wayne emerging with a sense of freedom in their lives, having gained from the experience and having good potential for the future. Wayne's growing comfort in his identity as an independent adult was evident in the interviews. During discussions over a two-year period he became much less concerned about the interviewer's response to him. He became more confident and comfortable with his sense of self.

The Variables in Wayne's Separation

Variable 1. The readiness of the individual for independence. Wayne's childhood was a steady progression toward independence. His parents' expectation was that he would increase his independence, and they openly expressed those feelings. Wayne's independence, they felt and obviously showed, was a sign of their success as parents. In that context, independence was safe to strive for within the relationship. Wayne was given the opportunity to experience ever-increasing independence as a child at a rate with which he dealt successfully. Independence was not thrust on him before he could handle it; he was provided with opportunities to handle independence successfully at a rate that responded to his needs-for example, going away from home for longer periods of time with the scout troups, going away to college and accepting more responsibility for budgeting his finances in college. The parents gave a clear message that Wayne was expected to be successful at handling independence and that independence was desirable.

Obviously, his parents also felt that they could handle the separation, although it was somewhat painful for them. They had a general optimism about their future. Mr. and Mrs. Marlie had a basic confidence in their adaptive abilities. Mrs. Marlie had many friends and interests. She had been able to work successfully prior to Wayne's being born, and she had plans to go back to work. As time went on, the parents talked about taking trips with each other. Mr. Marlie also had alternative outlets for his creativity. He was a successful businessman and craftsman. They felt very good about parenting, but they had outside interests. Both viewed Wayne's independence as a result of their being successful parents. This added to their self-esteem and feeling of confidence in being able to cope with life's tasks.

Another important aspect of their facing independence from Wayne was that Mr. and Mrs. Marlie got along well with each other for several years of marriage before Wayne was born. Their marriage was, therefore, not dependent on children for its success.

In conclusion, both Wayne and his parents had a basic confidence in their ability to be independent from each other. This feeling had been encouraged by some good experiences with independence.

Variable 2. Cognitive influences, including object constancy and the assimilative-accommodative modes of adaptation. Object constancy and object relations in the family were very good, a result of the parents' being consistent and caring models, which created in the family predictable patterns of behavior. The language ability within this family was at a high level, as was the ability for abstraction. This contributed to Wayne's being easily able to recognize and define for himself consistent patterns of behavior. As a result, Wayne was able to define his identity as distinct from that of his parents in many areas. His and his parents' arguments over belief systems can be seen as a process where Wayne and his parents defined their differences and therefore their separation.

Wayne exhibited the ability to integrate assimilative-accommodative modes of responding to challenging new situations. He has had, in his growth and development, a constant ability to master new situations successfullynursery school, grade school, Boy Scouts, athletics. Wayne was not put in situations so complex or chaotic that they were beyond his ability to master.

In the early stages of separation, he often used accommodative modes to excess in finding and proving that he was separated from his parents. For example, he adapted himself to a number of philosophical and moral codes, which he took on in their totality, without integrating them into his former outlook. However, as time went on and he became more capable of coping with the awareness that he was separated from his parents, he developed a more integrated world view that included an assimilation of viewpoint more consistent with his past history but that also accommodated some of his new experiences. Again, his career goal of law and anthropology reflected this integration. It reflected his earlier ideological commitment to a better social system. However, it was integrated with the more realistic awareness that in order to have impact on society one must gain some legitimate authority, such as becoming an expert in some specialized field.

Mr. and Mrs. Marlie had good object relations and object constancy. They were able to separate and verbalize their own needs as distinct from their child's. They were also able to separate clearly Wayne's need to be independent from their own ambivalence toward letting go. This was not an easy task, and at times there was some blurring of needs, such as the early arguments where the parents unconsciously made Wayne feel guilty for his disparate beliefs. However, for the most part they were conscious of their different needs.

Both Mr. and Mrs. Marlie had well-developed accommodative modes. This was seen in their recognizing accurately their son's changes in viewpoint while also recognizing the ways in which he was similar to them. Their shift to a more independent life-style involved a major change in the reality of life goals for themselves. Mrs. Marlie grew up with the belief that her value in life was to be a wife, mother, and homemaker. Mr. Marlie grew up believing that his value was to be husband, father, and provider. In order to let go, they had to accommodate to a new belief that added to the purpose of life, that of pursuing personal pleasures outside of the traditional roles. Their new plans and pursuits, in the second year of Wayne's interviews, reflected that shift in orientation. For example, the original purpose of their camping trips was for the family to have fun together. For them to continue to enjoy the trips that orientation had to change.

Variable 3. The nature of the parent-child relationship. The relationship was characterized by a basic sense of trust, and genuine concern for each family member as an individual. There was a basic sense of safety in the relationship, even when there was ambivalence and conflict. There was trust that things could be worked out. Indeed, the anger, ambivalence, and conflict expressed in the relationship were painful, but they were viewed as normal within the context of an ongoing relationship. Anger was clearly defined within the family as different from rejection.

Mr. and Mrs. Marlie felt comfortable in setting limits for Wayne as he was growing up and in loosening those limits as Wayne was able to take care of himself. They expected Wayne to be angry at times about the limit setting, to rebel against them, and to test out limits, but they still felt comfortable maintaining those limits as necessary for Wayne's good. They felt confident that Wayne's anger was transient. Wayne then felt secure in knowing there were limits.

Communication in the family was relatively open and verbal. Anger and conflicts were expressed in discussions and arguments. More subtle expressions of feeling were also picked up by the family members so that, although in this family as in all others, there was much unconscious interaction, their system of communication was relatively open and consistent. In general, the Marlie family displayed a basic sense of security within the relationship, which gave them strength to face the struggle that the separation process brought on.

Variable 4. The past experiences of the parents and the adolescent in separation. As stated previously, Wayne had many opportunities for positive experiences of separation, and he was fortunate in that he did not experience any traumatic separations that he was developmentally unequipped to handle. He had the experiences of going away to Cub Scout camp, Boy Scout camp, and college. He also had the experience of dealing with the death of the family cat, which, although sad, was, with family support, a developmental experience instead of a traumatic one. In response to his friend's departure in high school, he was able to acknowledge openly the sadness associated with the loss without feeling overwhelmed by it. He had a number of separation experiences that he learned from because he was well equipped to cope with them.

As stated previously, the most important past experience of separation that affects parents is their experience in separating from their own parents. Information on the adolescence of Mr. and Mrs. Marlie was sparse. Mrs. Marlie moved out of her parents' house and got married not long after high school. This was considered a natural course of events, and she maintained good relations with her parents. The separation process very obviously did not interrupt good relations with her parents; the process seemed to be completed successfully. Not long after high school graduation, Mr. Marlie went into the service. This was also seen as a natural development for someone of his age. In high school he appeared to have done some testing of limits, such as missing school on some occasions and other minor infractions. However, he and his parents maintained a basically good relationship with each other, and the separation process was seen by them as being a natural course of events.

Therefore, neither Mr. nor Mrs. Marlie's adolescent separation from their parents was a significantly disruptive experience, and it was probably a positive one.

Variable 5. The cultural influences on the separation process. Wayne's separation took place in the late 1960s and early 1970s, a period during which there was much peer group pressure for rebellion as a sign of independence. Wayne chose peers who reflected this as a way to support his own rebellion toward his parents and his parental surrogates, such as his teachers. Although there was a good deal of support for rebellion, most students in the Wright Institute study reported that they loved their families. College offered the opportunity to explore life-styles different from those of the parents in a safe, uncommitted way.

With no formal rites of passage provided by contemporary culture to help either Wayne or his parents in the separation process, Mr. and Mrs. Marlie saw few guidelines or cultural norms on how fast to give up control and on what kinds of things to do to guide the process of separation.

Mrs. Marlie obviously felt that there was considerable support for her redefining and recommitting herself. She found an opportunity to return to work and for alternative expressions of her creativity. The culture does support freedom for alternative expressions of creativity.

The cultural pluralism and the quick pace of cultural change in California during this time made the separation process more complex. Because of the wide variety of cultural styles, Wayne had more to compare with his parents middle-class life-style. The rapid rate of cultural change threw into greater question the relevance and value of the parents' style of living in today's changing world. As a result, Wayne's experimentation with life-styles was more diverse than that reported in Offer and Offer's (1975) Midwestern sample. Furthermore, the identification process was a result of an integration of the assimilated reality developed in Wayne's childhood under the primary influence of his parents and of the accommodation to the changes he perceived in the culture. The culture, then, made the separation process more stressful, while providing greater diversity of individual expression.

In conclusion, the variables affecting Wayne's separation from his parents were nearly all prognostically excellent. As a result, Wayne and his parents mastered the process well and developed new, more independent, and satisfying relationships. As individuals, they developed more satisfying options.

Part III
PATHOLOGICAL ADOLESCENT-PARENTAL SEPARATION

CHAPTER 10

The Borderline Syndrome:

Actually, the term "borderline" seems to be poorly chosen. Although some of the symptoms that characterize the borderline are seen in a more pronounced form in schizophrenics, there are also marked differences. The borderline syndrome is a stable response, usually developed at pubescence, related to the adolescent-parent separation. It is not, as the term suggests, a process on the way to or out of schizophrenia, but is a pathological response that is stable throughout the individual's life.

Although these individuals' childhoods are troubled and possibly stormy on occasion, they can often get along adequately at home and in the community during their childhood years. Their symptoms during these years are often not seen as pathological. As the symptoms are related to the individuation-separation process, it is most often the issues of adolescence that bring on the turmoil that ultimately brings the borderline adolescent to the attention of the mental health or juvenile justice establishments.

As the symptomatology is so pronounced, its development and manifestation are quite obvious and observable. A close scrutiny of the borderline syndrome should help develop further sensitivity to the major issues of adolescent separation in general. Many adolescents experience difficulties related to separating from parents, and many of these difficulties reflect some of the characteristics of the borderline syndrome. Very few of these adolescents, however, are considered borderline.

Oremland (1974), in "Three Hippies: A Study of Late-Adolescent Identity Formation," describes three adolescents who embraced the hippy identity for a while in search of an identity separate from that of their parents. All three lived for a time in a hippy community and exhibited similar behavior. All three saw Dr. Oremland in therapy because they were having problems. Only one, however, would be diagnosed as borderline, because he exhibited all, or nearly all, of the defining characteristics of the borderline. Furthermore, this individual was the only one who could not find a way out of the psychic pain he was experiencing; his difficulties remained.

In borderline individuals, all, or nearly all, of the variables that are related to the process of adolescent-parental separation represent inadequate preparation or have adverse experiences associated with them. With those individuals who develop borderline syndromes, only major therapeutic intervention will have a significant enough impact in helping them develop separate identities from their parents.

Characteristics of the Syndrome

The following description of the defining characteristics of the borderline syndrome is a synthesis of the characteristics most consistently reported by those noted for the study of the borderline: Burnham (1966), Deutsch (1942), Grinker et al. (1968), Gunderson et al. (1975), Gunderson and Singer (1975), Kernberg (1967), Knight (1953), Mahler (1968) Masterson (1972), Pfeiffer (1974), and Singer (1976). Mahler, Masterson, Gunderson, and Singer, have been especially concerned with pointing out the relationship of the descriptive and defining characteristics to the process of adolescent-parental separation. Bradley's study (1979) has added research evidence to the findings of clinical case studies reported by the others.

The affect of the borderline is generally dominated by feelings of freefloating anxiety, a feeling that something is wrong without knowing what it is. Borderlines often complain of a pervasive sense of emptiness, a detachment from feeling, and a general feeling that there is no reason to do anything in particular. Sometimes this is stated as being bored, as a general lack of enthusiasm, or as a lack of reason to do anything. After getting to know these individuals more deeply, one finds that the emptiness is, rather, a detachment from powerful feelings of depressive loneliness, what Masterson (1972) has defined as abandonment depression. Sporadically, rage comes out, directed toward others or themselves. These episodes often create further anxiety related to the fear of loss of control.

The prominent affects of the borderline generally reflect the affect associated with the early stages of bereavement. As with other bereavement processes, this affect produces considerable anxiety, and a tremendous amount of energy is directed at controlling it. However, unlike more healthy bereavement, in the borderline there is no attenuation of the feeling over time.

As stated previously, the development of the cognitive abilities of object constancy and object relations is an important variable in the separationindividuation process. In the borderline there is a deficiency in this development. This is usually a result of rather chaotic or contradictory object relations in the early years of life. This lack of ability to recognize consistency of behavior patterns makes it extremely difficult to observe role models accurately. It contributes to an inconsistent self-view. Under these circumstances even the self cannot be viewed with any object constancy; the self and others are seen as unpredictable.

These individuals, with their existential feelings of emptiness and lack of consistent self-view, were first described by Deutsch (1942). She referred to them as "as if personalities." She described a number of individuals who expressed concern over their lack of self-identity. They responded to this emptiness by taking on a role and acting as if they wanted to undertake the activities of the role, as well as expressing feelings that they thought were associated with the role. For example, a housewife would describe feelings that she believed to be appropriate but later would admit that she had none of these feelings.

These individuals lack a capacity for satisfaction and cannot find pleasure in any activity. If, for some reason, their opportunity to act out a role was disrupted, these individuals experienced severe personality disorganization. The related loneliness and depression would then emerge. They would, as quickly as possible, seek out another role to identify with, but again, their identification lacked related affect. In Eriksonian terms, there is a general identity diffusion, a lack of integration of the different components of the individual's personality, including discrepancy in his or her attitudes and affect and an absence of autonomy. Their behaviors, their feelings, and their attitudes are usually defined in reference to others either negatively or positively.

As stated in Part I, identity diffusion is a common component of the bereavement process when the separation disrupts the relationship with a significant other who has been used for defining the self, for example, a husband-wife relationship. This is seen especially in the separation between parent and adolescent, when the child is being redefined as an adult.

For the borderline, in whom the bereavement process is chronic and object relations underdeveloped, these issues are especially problematic. As a result, the individual must find some refuge from this emptiness and confusion. The refuge for many has been the "as if personality" described by Deutsch. Some of these individuals, occasionally and for brief periods, are flooded with powerful creative energy. It comes as if a dam had burst. They can often produce artistic works of high quality. However, because their creative activity comes only in spurts and because they are unable to sustain it, they usually derive little satisfaction and self-esteem from it. Under these circumstances, although creative activity provides some outlet for genuine affect, it cannot be identified with and is experienced as one more unintegrated, fragmented activity.

Their behavior varies from being able to function adequately in an environment to having very severe behavioral difficulties. The major variable that is operative is how structured the environment is and whether the environmental structure is explicit in a way in which they can understand with their diminished capacity for object constancy. When the environment is so structured, they can usually function adequately. When the environment lacks such structure and therefore must be created by the individual's implicit abilities, the borderline feels lost and his or her behavior may seem bizarre. The borderline therefore seems to have a propensity for getting into crises, either actual or felt.

This dependency on explicit structure probably is one of the reasons for the recent proliferation of observation and written material reflecting a greater concern with the borderline, as compared to when Deutsch first described this personality. The more relativistic and diverse the culture, the more dependent an individual must be on internal mechanisms for control and behavior patterns. This makes it more difficult for the borderline to get along. The "as if personality" gets along best in a structured environment with well-defined roles and social expectations.

In our present culture, unsupported by clear limits, the borderline's "as if personality" is a less effective defense against the powerful underlying affect and the associated fear of losing control. When there is a de-ruption of the continuity of their "roles," other defense mechanisms are used to avoid depression. The most prominent are denial, acting out, and object-splitting.

Their acting out includes a great deal of self-destructive behavior. This can be seen as an attempt to rid themselves of the abandonment depression by acting it out. The self-destructive behavior can include drug abuse, suicidal behavior, self-mutilation, sexual promiscuity, or sadomasochistic relationships. Sexual promiscuity often involves much older partners, who are sometimes homosexual, and usually ends with rejection by one or both parties. When describing their feelings associated with this acting out, they most often state that their reason for self-destructive behavior is that it gives them relief. That is, they feel that the anxiety and fear of losing control goes away after a self-destructive act. For example, after inflicting laceration, they suddenly feel very calm and good.

Object-splitting is a rather primitive defense mechanism to deal with feelings of ambivalence (Mahler 1975). Since object constancy is rather undeveloped, and since in the past, the borderline has been rejected for having negative feelings, ambivalence toward an individual seems unsafe. Anger has become tied to rejection. Therefore, those with whom the individual wants to be close are seen as all good. All negative feelings are projected onto other individuals. This sometimes alternates with one person being seen as all good at one time and as all bad at another. Further ambivalence that is self-directed is internalized in this manner, with the borderline at times seeing himself as all good, while at other times viewing himself as all bad. In this way he avoids rejection (separation) from one he cares about. For one so sensitive to separation, this is important to avoid.

No matter how well such individuals function outwardly, one difficulty that they frequently face is repeated nightmares. These become particularly bad when there is< external stress as well, which often causes a sleep disorder. These individuals, when faced with overwhelming environmental stress such as a major separation in their life or a disruption in the continuity of their "role," may suffer a brief psychotic episode. Pfeiffer (1974) defines these as "mini-psychoses," which usually last anywhere from minutes to several days. The onset is usually acute, and the re-compensation (cessation of psychotic symptoms) is equally quick. Return to a structured setting can be very helpful during these periods. Sometimes a powerful exhibition of their defense mechanisms can help them re-compensate. For example, individuals who are in the midst of a psychotic episode might do something selfdestructive, which can bring them back to a better feeling of control of themselves. The sleep disturbance, the psychotic behavior, and the disturbance in the thought processes subside.

The most dominant interpersonal aspect is the highly ambivalent relations with parents, especially the mother. The attitude toward this relationship usually vacillates between urges to cling to the mother or to reject her completely. These individuals intermittently develop other highly ambivalent relationships, which reflect the relationships they have with their parents.

As Burnham (1966) points out, borderline individuals are searching to reestablish an infantile relationship with an omnipotent, all-caring mother figure. They evoke, between themselves and this individual, what Burnham calls "the bargain"; if the mother figure provides for their needs for a while, they will be able to face the issues necessary for them to become their "ideal self." This "appeal," as Burnham calls it, often evokes feelings in the other individual of being the omnipotent helper. This helper is told that he or she is the only one capable of having this special relationship and that only he or she can save the other person. Other individuals involved in the borderline individual's milieu are often seen as a threat to this relationship and are the focus of all the negative projections.

The expectations of this relationship are unrealistic. Furthermore, the attitude toward it is ambivalent, since the person wants separation as well as attachment. Therefore, it ultimately ends in disappointment for both individuals involved and often causes bitterness on both sides.

This ambivalence toward separation once again reflects the dynamics of the first and second stages of bereavement. However, the repetitive projection of this ambivalence on to third parties continually serves to enable the borderline to avoid the issues with the primary party, the parents.

Often the individual also has a large number of superficial, transient relationships. These relationships usually give some gratification without causing much anxiety.

Singer (Gunderson and Singer 1975) has reported characteristic profiles of the borderline syndrome on psychological testing, and her findings are consistent with the preceding discussion. She found that on structured tests such as the Bender-Gestalt and WAIS, there is no particular deviation from the norm, with some individuals attaining quite high scores. On more projective tests such as the Rorschach and T.A.T., they show unique creativity, while their stories are markedly hostile with depressive content. They also show some bizarre content, not unlike that of schizophrenics. Singer points out, however, that unlike schizophrenics, they recognize the bizarre response. For example, after stating something bizarre, they will say, "That was pretty weird." This self-observing ego is generally lacking in the schizophrenic.

In conclusion, the feelings of anxiety, fear, rage, depression, and loneliness are those associated with the early periods of bereavement. The lack of a capacity for pleasure and identity diffusion are further issues of the bereavement process. Highly ambivalent feelings toward the mother, undeveloped object-constancy and object-relations, and a lack of preparedness for separation all combine to make the adolescent unable to deal with the issues of adolescent-parental separation and force him to develop a defensive style to avoid it. The result is an individual stuck in the process.

CHAPTER 11

Case History of Greg Davis

Greg Davis is nineteen years old, and he is a borderline adolescent. He was born in Minneapolis, the second of three boys. He looks his age, is tall and thin, and, when not feeling unduly depressed, would be considered goodlooking.

The Childhood Environment

When Greg was born, his father had recently attained a middlemanagement position in a large food industry corporation, and the family lived in an upper-middle-class area. Evidently they were well-respected members of the community. The father, following Greg's birth, continued to be upwardly mobile in his company until he became vice-president, when Greg was ten. The family then moved to a high socio-economic area.

Financial and social status have always been the most prominent, overt goals of the family. Both parents have been involved in community affairs to further enhance the family's status in the community.

Greg's Mother

Mrs. Davis met Mr. Davis while in college, and they were married after a one-year courtship. Mrs. Davis dropped out to help Mr. Davis through school. She was a good student but evidently had no regrets about leaving school. She has relied primarily on the family's social status for her own self-esteem.

Following Mr. Davis's graduation from college, Mrs. Davis became pregnant with the first of their sons. After this, there was a ten-year period in which the family was forced to move a number of times because Mr. Davis's upward mobility in the company caused repeated transfers to new areas.

When the family became somewhat settled again, Greg was born. Greg stated that his mother told him that she had been hoping for a girl at the time. Mrs. Davis became pregnant about two years later, again with the desire of having a girl. Greg's youngest brother was born in 1957, when Greg was 2 ½ years old.

Mrs. Davis was quite compulsive, especially in her housekeeping; she demanded that her house be immaculate, especially if guests were expected.

Mrs. Davis rarely verbalized emotion, either positive or negative. The only exception to this was during periods of heavy intoxication. These varied in frequency during different periods of Greg's life, ranging from once or twice a week to once a month. Mr. and Mrs. Davis often got drunk together. While intoxicated, they would frequently become extremely enraged at one another, sometimes striking each other or throwing things. Mr. Davis would do the most damage and then would feel guilty the following day. With the exception of an occasional bruise, these incidents never caused any physical injury.

Mrs. Davis overtly dominated the family. The rules for the children, as well as the other decisions that affected the whole family-for example, where to go on vacation-were nearly always made by her. Her domination was not generally by overt authoritarian dictates, but rather by feeling righteously indignant and hurt if others disagreed with her. It was difficult for family members to confront her on this, because she genuinely felt that all her decisions were for the "good of the family," and she always put the "good of the family" before herself. Furthermore, the family feared the mother's not being in control. Such a change would create a major upset of the family homeostasis. The family feared that if the mother did not provide control, no one else would.

Food was a central issue for her and the family. According to Greg, she was an excellent cook. She cooked large meals and felt rejected if the family did not partake of them in large quantities. As a result, all the members of the family were overweight, except Greg. Greg, referring to his mother's use of food in the family, stated: "My mother equated giving food with giving love, but to me it was only her trying to control us. I saw through this at an early age ... sometimes I used to dream that my mother was trying to swallow me."

The contrast in body image, with Greg being skinny and the rest of the family being fat, reflected a general family view that Greg was deviant from the rest. This attitude was mutually held by Greg and his family. In childhood he was called headstrong by family members; at pubescence this concept changed to his being seen as sick.

Up to this point, Greg had been the only member of the family to rebel overtly against the mother's control. A large part of his rebellion was covertly encouraged by the family. In this sense, the family used him by projecting onto him their own rebellious feelings toward the mother's control. Even the mother used him for this purpose, projecting much of her own ambivalence and guilt about her control onto him. In a nonverbal way she essentially was saying, "I expect someone to rebel against this control." The fear of the mother not being in control, however, was much too great for this message to be dealt with consciously by any family member. Greg's rebellious behavior, although covertly encouraged, overtly had to be seen as outside the limits of behavior allowable by the other family members. Thus, Greg's behavior was labeled sick. Furthermore, these important issues within the family were only communicated nonverbally by the acting out of the feelings. Mother, in describing Greg's history, stated that he was different from her other children almost from birth. He was not cuddly and affectionate and became even less so as he grew older. She said that he had, in fact, been "sick" for a long time. She found it necessary to repeat several times during our conversations that she had been a good mother to him and that his brothers had "turned out just fine"—one was already a very successful businessman. Several times she stated that she was very concerned about Greg's welfare and would do anything that she could but that she had no desire to interfere with the therapist's "treatment of him."

Greg expressed strong feelings toward his mother, alternating between loving feelings and hostility. At times he would see his mother as loving him and would take full responsibility for their not getting along, even when a child. He commented that he used to cause his mother so much trouble that she had neck pains. He once brought up, in a bragging style but with a vigilant look at the therapist's response, that his mother would sometimes walk around the house in her underwear when her husband was not home. On further questioning, he seemed uncertain about what to make of this behavior. He seemed to feel both sexually aroused and guilty about it, and he felt controlled and angry at his mother. At other times Greg would see her as cold and rejecting, as never allowing him any privacy or freedom, as never allowing him to ask her questions as a child, and as liking the other boys more.

During the interview, when his mother was discussed, Greg would often express murderous rage. The rage was nearly always followed by a disavowal of it and by guilt associated with the feelings.

In conversations, Mrs. Davis expressed mixed messages toward her son's treatment. She stated that she had no desire to interfere, then followed this immediately by telling the therapist how to view Greg. She stated further that she would do anything to assist in the treatment, and then implied that all such effort was doomed to failure.

An assessment of these conversations was that consciously Mrs. Davis was concerned for her son and desired change, but unconsciously she was quite fearful of having her son improve. This unconscious fear had three possible sources, the first being fear of rejection by a "healthy son." (Rejection from a sick son could be discounted as sick behavior.) Second, if her son was able to function well in society as a result of treatment, she would feel responsible for his earlier difficulties rather than being able to blame them on some unexplained, unalterable evil influence such as "mental illness." Finally, a healthy son would undermine the family myth that rebellion against mother was "sick," and the mother, as well as the rest of the family, feared this loss of control.

Greg's Father

When Mr. and Mrs. Davis met, he was working part-time and attending college part-time as a business major. Following their marriage, because Mrs. Davis was working, Mr. Davis was able to reduce his working hours and attend college full-time.

Upon graduation, Mr. Davis was made a foreman at the plant where he had been working. He was an extremely assertive, hard-working, and dedicated employee, often putting in longer hours than expected. Mr. Davis was promoted rapidly. Each time he had a new position, he was able to distinguish himself and to win new promotions.

Mr. Davis appeared to have been rather distant from his family. As a result of his work, he often spent long periods away from them. He also was involved in a number of civic projects, which further taxed his time and energy.

Another distancing factor was a number of affairs that Mr. Davis had throughout the history of his marriage. These were never discussed by family members except when they were mentioned as part of a drunken argument between Mr. and Mrs. Davis. During these arguments, Mr. Davis would often accuse Mrs. Davis of having affairs, but she continually denied these allegations. Greg believed that his mother did not have affairs, although he was quite aware of his father's.

Mr. Davis's relationship to the family was rather distant and aloof, but he was submissive to his wife. For the most part, he went along with whatever she felt was for the good of the family. Mr. Davis was very authoritarian with his children. As Mrs. Davis put it, "he took no sass from them." His main overt relationship with his children was that of the heavy disciplinarian, relying on both corporal punishment and the removal of privileges for the children's transgressions. These punishments were usually given at the request of Mrs. Davis, or when Mr. Davis became angry at the children. When Mr. Davis did spend time with his children, his demeanor, according to Greg, was unpredictable. He was at times warm and friendly and at other times cold and critical. Greg felt that his father's criticism was most often directed at him.

Of obvious importance to Mr. Davis was social status. He often told his children of his successes on the football field and encouraged them to follow in his footsteps. The eldest son, John, had played football in high school, and Mr. Davis was quite proud of this.

Greg stated that he felt that he had spent his whole life trying to please his father, but to no avail. He took most pride in his musical abilities and often tried to get his father's approval. His father continually ignored these attempts and sometimes disparaged his musical abilities.

When Greg was seventeen, his father had a severe heart attack. Convalescence took about six months, after which Mr. Davis returned to work. Six months later he had another heart attack and died.

Greg angrily refused numerous attempts to discuss his feeling regarding the loss of his father. He stated flatly that it was best not to discuss it, that it had no effect on him, and that therefore he would not talk about it. It seemed unwise to press the matter before Greg was ready to talk about it, so little discussion regarding his father took place until considerable time had passed.

Greg's Siblings

There were no psychiatric histories of either of Greg's two siblings. They were considered by the family to be quite healthy and, on the whole, "good" boys.

John, the oldest child in the family and ten years Greg's senior, was evidently Mr. Davis's favorite. He did moderately well in school. Although overweight, he played football in high school with some success. He graduated from college and was the owner-operator of a small, successful business.

Greg had his ups and downs in his relationship with John. Evidently, he always felt jealous because of his older brother's favored status with his father.

Tony, 2 ½ years younger than Greg, was the favorite of Mrs. Davis. Greg referred to him as a "momma's boy" and said that he was spoiled. Tony has done well in school. At last report, he was living at home and planning to go to college.

Greg had his ups and downs with Tony also. Tony was his favorite family member, although he stated that he did not have close or strong feelings for Tony.

The sibling rivalry among the three boys was quite strong. As has been indicated, both John and Tony earned much greater recognition for their achievements in business and in school than Greg was able to earn for his talents in music.

Greg's Past History

Mrs. Davis stated that her pregnancy with Greg was normal and that he was full term. Greg's birth was without complication. He was a healthy infant and had, on the whole, a healthy childhood. Developmental milestones were within normal limits.

Mrs. Davis stated that Greg was not a "cuddly baby," and became even less so while still quite young. Greg stated that he did not remember his mother touching him very much and that he really did not like his mother to touch him.

When Tony was born, Mrs. Davis stated that she "could not handle both children" and sent Greg to nursery school for most of the day. In preparation for this, his toilet training was rather abruptly completed soon after she became pregnant.

Greg had several memories from between ages six and eight that stood out. He remembered that Tony often got candy when he cried and that he never received any. As a result, he started stealing the candy from his brother, threatening to hit him if he told his parents. He remembered being quite frightened when his mother and father got into fights while drunk. He recalled wanting to rescue his mother. After one of these fights he went into the bathroom, saw a razor blade, and cut his finger until it bled. He could not remember any reason for the self-destructiveness, and this was the only selfdestructive behavior he remembered prior to pubescence.

Christmas, Greg said, was always a pleasant time of year for him as a child. His parents were usually nice to him, and he would receive nice gifts.

A tragedy occurred when he was ten—the family dog was killed by an automobile. He felt close to the dog but remembered times when he had alternately petted the dog and hit him. He felt responsible for the dog's death for no logical reason and felt very guilty about the way he had treated the dog.

When Greg was ten he began taking piano lessons from an older woman. He stated that this woman had cared about him more than any other person had, and although he had to stop taking lessons when he was twelve because he started getting into trouble and lived away from home, he maintained occasional contact with her.

Greg did adequately in grammar school, although he got into trouble on several occasions—for example, he was sent home for getting into fights with other children and for disobedience several times. Greg's fights were almost always with children who were bigger than he was, and he nearly always got the worst of it. On the whole his academic record in grammar school was average but with As in music.

It was around the age of twelve that Greg began acting "antisocial" to a degree that motivated his parents and school to seek psychiatric help. This behavior included keeping company with the "wrong crowd," drug use, and disobedience at home and at school. Greg stated that he began lying to his parents a lot "to keep them off my back." "He cut school most of the time and began using drugs, primarily marijuana. At times his parents responded by ignoring the transgressions and by being more lenient, while at other times they were very strict and punitive.

Greg stated that his parents began blaming him for everything negative that happened in the family, such as arguments between mother and father and other family discord. He was set up as the bad example who was not to be trusted around his younger brother, for fear of his "bad" influence.

The family sought psychiatric help for Greg when he was twelve. From that point on, Greg was under continuous psychiatric treatment. He was placed in a private psychiatric hospital shortly after treatment began. The reasons given for the hospitalization were his inability to get along at home, his antisocial behavior at school, and drug abuse.

During the next three years, he was sent to a number of live-in private schools for emotionally disturbed children and was hospitalized for several short periods. The hospitalizations occurred when the staff at the school facilities felt that his acting out behavior was beyond their control. This behavior included getting into fights, drug abuse, defiance of rules and authority figures, and cutting himself, as well as other self-destructive behaviors.

Greg was seen to be quite different in one-to-one interactions. He was, at these times, regarded as friendly, thoughtful, considerate, and helpful to others more disturbed than himself.

At fifteen, he was sent for long-term hospitalization to a private hospital in the South, several hundred miles from home. He stayed at this hospital for approximately two years.

Greg's psychiatrist at the hospital stated that he had been a very difficult patient to treat. He was seen by the staff as a manipulating sociopath at one time and as a very sick child at another. In response to this split in behavior, some staff members mothered him, while others were very authoritarian and punitive with him.

He had a number of brief psychotic episodes, during which he became paranoid and fearful of losing control. During one of these episodes he became violent, breaking a psychiatric technician's nose. These psychotic episodes usually lasted less than an hour, after which Greg felt guilty and ashamed of his behavior. At other times Greg was well controlled and was very cooperative and productive. At times he appeared to be severely depressed.

Greg had difficulty getting along with most of his peers. He would make a friend for a while but would soon break off the relationship, usually with some angry confrontation and expressions of distrust.

The one exception to this was a friendship Greg made with a girl who he continued to feel close to even after several years. She was evidently discharged from the hospital not long before he was. The duration of their relationship, however, was only a month long. Therefore, it is probable that the importance of this relationship had grown in Greg's memory.

Because of the acute onset and recompensation of Greg's psychotic episodes, a seizure disorder was suspected. A complete neurological workup was done at the hospital. The neurologist's report stated that no abnormalities showed up on the electroencephalogram, but he felt the results were inconclusive.

While at the hospital, Greg was treated with a range of medications, primarily major tranquilizers and antiseizure medication. His attending physician during this hospitalization felt that these medications were helpful, although symptom relief was only minor at best. Greg's violent episode with the psychiatric technician resulted in his termination from this hospital, and he was sent to the state hospital. The doctor stated that the state hospital provided firmer structure and that Greg responded with better self-control. He was soon sent home, under the care of his psychiatrist.

Greg's attitude toward returning home was highly ambivalent. On a number of occasions while hospitalized he had made plans for returning home. He would then sabotage the plans, often blaming the staff for his not being able to go home.

Within six months of Greg's return home, his father died of a heart attack. Soon after this he ran away from home and started roaming around the Midwest and the South. He returned home intermittently, never staying long. About nine months prior to our initial meeting, Greg agreed to work for his brother's firm on the West Coast.

Greg stated that he and his brother got along only for a brief period after his arrival and that he left the job and began "living on the streets." He described his occupation since coming to San Francisco as "street hustler." This entailed living in crash pads and eating and sleeping irregularly. His income, he stated, was from pan handling, drug dealing, and occasionally playing piano in a bar. The latter is questionable since although he does have the musical ability, he is underage and looks it.

Since coming to San Francisco he has used drugs quite heavily and indiscriminately, using, as he puts it, "Whatever I can get my hands on."

While in San Francisco he made no friends, although he had many acquaintances. He further stated that he got into frequent fights, always with men larger than himself, and he often got beat up.

He had been hospitalized in the city twice prior to the hospitalization in which I met him. Both were the result of self-destructive behavior—selfinflicted lacerations—and drug abuse. Following the first hospitalization he went to a half-way house, where he stayed only a few days. He left after two days, against medical advice, the last time he was hospitalized.

When feeling acutely depressed he often used emergency psychiatric facilities; however, he was unwilling or unable to follow through on any longterm program.

The day of admission to the hospital and our first meeting, Greg said that he woke up feeling as though no one cared about him. He went to one emergency' room asking for a pain-killer for leg pain. Known to personnel there as a drug abuser, he was refused. He then went to another emergency room, where he told them he was severely agitated and suicidal. He was given a major tranquilizer, enough for three days, at which time he was supposed to have a follow-up appointment. He then went to a busy intersection, took all the medication, and proceeded to cut himself with broken glass to prove "that no one cared." Following this, he went back to the first emergency room, where he walked around with his cut arms as evidence of their disregard for him. After about fifteen minutes, he states, "someone noticed me."

He told the doctor on call that he would either kill himself at the bridge or cut his throat if he was not admitted. Immediately after admission he asked to be discharged and was put on a seventy-two-hour hold.

Greg's Behavior on the Psychiatric Unit:

When Greg came into the inpatient unit about an hour after he had been referred from the emergency room, he was rather drowsy from the medication he had taken a few hours earlier. The initial intake interview was postponed until morning.

In the morning, Greg appeared for his interview in what looked like moderately priced casual clothing-slacks and a sport shirt-which appeared not to have been cleaned in some time. He was tall and gangly, and he looked his nineteen years. He affected a tough-guy manner but was obviously anxious and fearful. He talked very loudly during the initial interview. His body looked like a battlefield. There were cuts, scrapes, and bruises everywhere, including lacerations completely covering both arms, although none severe enough to require stitches.

He talked extremely fast and had difficulty sitting still. He had broad mood swings during the interview, appearing at times depressed and suicidal, while at other times angry and threatening-for example, "I'll leave right now; you can't keep me." At still other times, he appeared to be fearfully hypervigilant, and at still others, like the ideal patient. He was quite manipulative during the interview. He said all the things that get one hospitalized, while at the same time he threatened to leave. He obviously wanted hospitalization without asking for it. He stated that at times he was fearful of losing control, that he had felt a buildup of anger recently, and that no one cared about him. At the same time he said that he had been offered a $50,000 contract to play piano for a musical group, that he could become a doctor if he wished, and that he knew more about psychology than the therapist.

Greg stated that he had brief periods when he lost control, which were preceded by olfactory hallucinations. He said he had had a workup for epilepsy but that the findings were negative. He was obviously anxious during discussion of his loss of control. He further stated that he had had racing thoughts recently and could not slow down. His appetite and sleep pattern, he said, were irregular-at times good, at other times bad. He wanted medication but would not take phenothiazines (class of major tranquilizer); he wanted something similar to help him slow down. Obviously he had picked up a great deal of medical and psychological knowledge, although some was incorrect. Results of a formal mental status examination showed orientation, abstract abilities, calculations, long- and short-term memory, and general information to be within normal limits.

He reported no history of hallucinations except the olfactory ones previously described. Greg ended the intake interview by stating that he did not want any relatives notified of his hospitalization.

Greg was regarded by the nursing staff on the ward as a difficult patient almost from the moment he arrived. He was hyperactive, manipulative, loud, demanding, and always testing the limits. He was admitted on a seventy-twohour hold as "a danger to himself," and he stated that he would leave when it was up and kill himself. He was constantly demanding medication for a host of somatic complaints and became angry when he was refused.

Group therapy was an anxious time for him, especially the first two days. After each of his first two groups, he ran out of the hospital and appeared to have brief psychotic episodes, lasting about half an hour. On both occasions staff followed him, and he threatened to attack anyone who came close to him. He appeared paranoid, mistaking any approach as an attack. On both occasions his therapist was called. At first his behavior was threatening; only after being reassured that no one was going to hurt him and that he needed help that could be provided did he return. After returning to the ward on both occasions, he pronounced the way he had just acted as crazy, stating that he did not know what had come over him. He was able to remember the events of the episode in general but not in detail.

On the third day of hospitalization he signed in as a voluntary patient. The following day, a marked change in his behavior occurred. His new behavioral pattern remained stable until discharge.

He took on the role of ideal patient in relation to the staff. In relation to the other patients, he acted, at times, as a leader, and at other times, rather detached.

During this period in psychotherapy, he related many dreams and talked of needing to change and of working hard, of his failures in the past, and of his past history-all the things psychotherapists like to hear. He did not appear to be relating this information because he felt it was important. He was quite obviously trying to interest and please the therapist and genuinely seemed to want to develop a relationship. He expected that pleasing the therapist was the way to do it. This rather seductive behavior was characteristic of his manipulative style, which he used in his attempts to gain acceptance from those with whom it appeared he desired some social contact and intimacy.

Some issues discussed in therapy appeared to have some importance to him. For example, his grandiose claims were discussed in terms of his expectation that he must be something that he considered superior in order to be accepted and that therefore he could not commit himself to anything real. He discussed his loneliness and his dissatisfaction with relating to people on a very superficial level, devoid or separated from his feelings. For example, he stated once, "You'll marry a nurse one day, and after I make it in music, I'll marry a groupie." His statement that doctors marry nurses and musicians marry groupies reflects his view that people are primarily motivated by playing roles devoid of feeling.

Although issues such as these were discussed, the affectual investment that accompanied them was usually strongly defended against.

In group therapy Greg remained extremely anxious, having numerous excuses for needing to leave, such as somatic complaints. When he did stay, he attempted to keep attention focused on himself, either by giving advice to other patients or by confessing his difficulties. After a confession he wanted to be rewarded with lauds of bravery for his opening up. He found it very difficult to share attention and felt rejected when confronted on this point.

In the second week of hospitalization, Greg appeared to be in better control; his mood had elevated, and he no longer felt suicidal. Discharge plans were begun.

Greg was in need of a place to live where his manipulation would be confronted and limits would be set on his behavior, while at the same time the staff would be tolerant of him and would provide opportunity for positive relationships to develop. He was accepted into a local halfway house. In compliance with their requirement to have a daily activity, he found volunteer work at a free clinic. It was suggested to him that this would put him into close contact with people whom he had previously dealt drugs. He insisted that this was the job he wanted, his reason being that this was an opportunity for him to prove that he was a changed person.

During the days just prior to his discharge, he appeared to regress somewhat, feeling more depressed and being more manipulative. On several occasions he threatened to check out against medical advice and to reject all his discharge plans. He declared during these periods that he was off to become a famous musician. In psychotherapy he could not relate his changes in behavior to any change in feelings, and he rejected all suggestions that it could be related to his discharge plans.

During the final day of his hospitalization, Greg described a dream he had had that was depressing him. He related, while sobbing, that the dream was based on real events that had occurred following a previous hospitalization. The dream, he said, was like reliving it as it had really happened. The dream involved the girl with whom he had been close in the previous hospitalization. He said that, although she was five years older than him, he had loved her and had never wanted to leave her. As previously stated, he had gone from the private hospital to a state hospital for several months. During this period, the girl had been discharged to her home in Texas.

In the dream, after he had been discharged, he hitchhiked to her home; upon arriving, he found that she had died of "unknown causes." His associations to the dream were primarily mystical feelings that she would return and that they could be reunited.

He rejected an interpretation that connected his despair and fear of separation in the dream to his fears of separation from his present hospitalization—a fear of losing contact with people with whom he had become close during the hospitalization.

Greg's Behavior in the Group Home:

Greg's behavior in the group home was similar to his behavior in the hospital. There were markedly differing reactions to Greg among the staff. Some felt very close to Greg and saw him as a child, while others saw him as a manipulating, self-centered brat. At times he threatened to leave, while at other times he demanded their attention.

When Greg became depressed he often acted out self-destructively, such as by cutting himself and using drugs. Rules of the house were continually being tested, and on several occasions Greg almost got kicked out.

Soon after starting his volunteer job, he began missing work, stating that he was just too depressed to go. As a result, he entered a structured day program, which, although he continually complained about it, he attended fairly regularly. This program included daily group therapy, wood shop, community meeting, and a recreational activity.

When Greg first came to the halfway house, his peer relations were similar to those that he had had in the hospital. He isolated himself from the rest of the residents. At times he would become sociable in order to develop some closeness with a new resident for a few days, and then he would find some fault with the person and break off the relationship. Usually Greg was the dominant person in the relationship, and it was based on the other person's rapidly developing a strong dependence on him. He would try to be, for this person, everything he wished someone would be for him. This quickly became intolerable for both parties, and the relationship soon ended.

Now, a year after entering the group home, a great deal has changed. Greg has developed two relationships that he feels are important to him. One of these relationships has lasted several months already. It is quite different from past relationships in that it is neither casual nor based on a strong dependency need of either person but involves fairly equal give and take.

Greg states that he has not stolen anything for quite some time. This change seems to be related to a new-found ability to identify with his peers "You just can't steal from people as needy as you are."

He has also become compulsive about telling the truth. He says, "I never lie anymore. You can't like yourself if you can't feel another person can accept you for what you really are. If I tell the truth and someone doesn't like it, fuck them."

When Greg's mood is up, he remains quite busy. He attends his day program regularly and has taken a two-hour-a-week gardening job. He practices his music sporadically, is writing poetry, and has taken a keen interest in reading psychology textbooks.

Greg still suffers severe depressive periods. These periods appear less frequently and he remains in better control during them, but he becomes extremely frustrated, fearing he is doing no better. Symptoms still include fear of losing control, social withdrawal, sleep disorder, psychomotor retardation, anxiety, paranoid ideation, and self-destructive acting out. Symptoms appear to be less severe than a year ago. For the most part, these depressive periods seem to be related to social rejection, either past, present, or anticipated.

Greg is presently transferring from his halfway house to another because of a residency time limit. Although he has been depressed as a result of this change, he has been able to connect the feeling with the reasons for it. He states that he has never left anywhere before on good terms, and this time he is determined to leave in a good way.

During the past year Greg has, on several occasions, attempted to make contact with his mother. This has usually been during times when he has felt least angry at her, and when he has felt in the most control. His mother has been generally unresponsive to him.

As can be seen, in the past year much has changed for Greg.

The Course of Greg's Psychotherapy

The main goal that Greg and the therapist have set out in psychotherapy is to develop a relationship that is as open and honest as possible, in which communication is as verbal as possible, and that allows for dependency needs while still allowing for individuality. The goal is a relationship that is continuous and stable, while at the same time *slowly* moving from Greg's being very dependent on the therapist to ever-increasing autonomy. In other words, it is an attempt to establish a close but non-symbiotic relationship from which it is safe to explore individuality. The process is creating an attachment between patient and therapist from which the process of separation can occur in a positive developmental way. If Greg can learn to separate from the therapist in a safe way, it is hoped that he can apply these experiences toward other separations, especially to psychological separation from his parents. At the outset of the relationship, the therapist took the greater responsibility for formulating and expressing these goals, while encouraging Greg to accept more of the responsibility.

In the past year this process has occurred in part, but it is in no way complete. This relationship is in such sharp contrast to his other important relationships that it has been extremely difficult to maintain this constancy. It has, however, become somewhat easier to maintain this direction as time goes on.

Although many issues such as day-to-day activities, mood swings, past history, philosophy of life, and interpersonal relations have been discussed through the course of psychotherapy, the center focus has continuously been the dynamics of this relationship. If this is not continuously dealt with, the communication inevitably becomes acted out in another way rather than verbalized.

In the beginning of this relationship, Greg was highly ambivalent towards the therapist. When he went to the group home, his initial behavior continued to alternate between being a seductive "ideal patient" and being rejecting and hostile. He wanted the therapist to be a completely nourishing and omnipotent figure, while at the same time he wanted complete subservience. During this stage of the relationship, misunderstandings of anything Greg said enraged him; he said that he was all alone. He took any frustration of his wishes as a sign of rejection and conversely expected rejection continuously. He was continually testing limits in these areas.

"What if I broke your office window?" he would ask.

"I would be angry, I would demand that you pay for it, but I would continue to want to work with you."

In the early period of treatment he once acted this out by breaking a flower pot. He was angry at having to pay for it but could hardly believe that the therapist still wanted to work with him—he was greatly reassured. The reason for making him pay for the pot was to give him the message that he could take adult responsibility; paying also helped relieve his guilt and demonstrated the therapist's reliability.

As the attachment has strengthened, Greg has been able to derive increased security from it and has begun to accept some feelings of dependency. As the importance of the relationship increased, he became more and more fearful of being rejected or deserted. Besides seeing the therapist twice weekly, Greg called him at home once or twice a week for several months, wanting reassurance. After he had heard the assurance of concern for him, he would sometimes challenge the therapist to come to see Kim. On these occasions, however, interaction was limited to the phone. For the most part, he would feel reassured from the telephone conversations, and usually remarked later that he had felt better after the talk.

This behavior has attenuated, although if he feels angry or rejected by the therapist or anyone else, the need for reassurance is again stimulated.

Another reflection of Greg's move from a desire for uncontrolled closeness to a more comfortable acceptance of realistic closeness is an attenuation of fearful homosexual fantasies toward the therapist. During early interviews Greg made a number of references to feelings that the therapist must be homosexual to take such an interest in him. He had difficulty at that point in separating sexuality from closeness, as well as in integrating sexuality with closeness. He has recently made few accusations about the therapist's being homosexual, and he feels more understanding of the separation of sexuality from interest in him.

Greg recently brought up a new topic of discussion. He stated that in time he may want to see another psychotherapist, with whom he can start out on an "adult level." He said he does not, however, want to give up his dependency on his current therapist and that he wants to continue with both at the same time. This has introduced direct discussions of the conflict concerning becoming independent, thus giving up the dependency relationship and being able to attain the rewards and self-esteem of an adultto-adult relationship. Greg stated that he does not feel ready to give up this psychotherapeutic relationship yet, but someday he is going to want to. However, he wants an understanding that he can return if he feels the need. This realization that he can separate without destroying the relationship is a new way of looking at things for him.

Following these discussions he has experienced feelings of depression. Unlike past depressive periods, however, this depression has been felt openly and is verbally expressed with relatively little self-destructive acting out.

Another aspect of Greg's separation from his therapist has been a greater comfort in his being critical of the therapist without experiencing undue anxiety, as well as his feeling somewhat competitive with the therapist—for example, disagreeing with an interpretation that has been made or feeling that an interpretation that he has made is better. This behavior has been strongly supported and interpreted as his learning to do for himself those things that the therapist previously did for him.

Concurrent to these discussions Greg is in the process of separating from his halfway house and is doing this more positively than he has in any previous separation.

In relation to his mother, Greg has gained greater control over his acting out in reference to his feelings toward her and has become somewhat open about discussing the relationship. For a long while, his discussions of Mrs. Davis, like those he had in the hospital, were primarily limited to brief outbursts of either rage or hurt toward her, often followed by a denial of the previous affect. Usually the attempt to follow up on these outbursts was met by refusals to talk about it further. Once when it was suggested that he sounded hurt and angry about his mother's rejection of him, he ran out of the room swearing. The next hour he began by stating that he was angry at the therapist for taking unfair control over the discussion and that he was not ready to discuss "those things." Greg has become somewhat more comfortable talking about his parents' treatment of him.

At different times Greg has talked for brief periods regarding his feeling toward his mother. He has stated that his ultimate wish is for his mother to love and accept him for what he is. He used to think that this could happen, but now he believes that it probably will not. He has stated on occasion that he still fantasizes that she will call him up, tell him she loves him, and ask him to come home; he really knows, however, that this will not happen. Greg still hopes that someday his mother will want to be friends or at least have some positive contact with him. It makes him sad that his mother is not close to him, but now, unlike the past, he believes that he can live without her. He still has angry outbursts toward his mother and feels hopeless because of his feeling toward her, but these periods are becoming rarer.

Greg still says very little regarding his present feelings toward his father. He has, however, stated that in some ways his therapist is more of a father to him than he has ever had.

In conclusion, Greg has made important strides in facing the issues of his separation from his parents, but he is still far from resolving them.

CHAPTER 12

Discussion of Greg Davis's Separation from His Parents

The most prominent characteristics of Greg Davis's interpersonal, intrapsychic, affective, and behavioral life are generally shared by those who are regarded as borderline personalities. The importance of this to our discussion of adolescent separation is not that individuals with shared characteristics can be found but that the characteristics fit together into a recognizable pattern. The patterns, as with Greg, generally develop during pubescence and remain largely stable for the rest of the life cycle. These patterns develop in adolescence, as with Greg, in individuals who have a similar background; the most outstanding characteristics are a mother who is ambivalent about her child's becoming individuated from her and who does not feel safe unless she is in control of the family and a father who is also ambivalent toward the control of the mother and deals with this by psychologically distancing himself and being aloof within the family (Masterson 1972). The father's ambivalent feelings are projected onto the adolescent.

The characteristics that developed in Greg, and that are generally shared by the borderline, are those of an individual caught in a continual state of pathological separation. On the one hand, he is motivated to separate by biological and cultural forces that are pushing him toward adult status and responsibility, but on the other hand, he fears separation because of the inadequate preparation and poor experiences associated with attempts to separate and individuate in childhood. This has resulted in Greg's being in a continual state of ambivalence toward separation and therefore a continual state of bereavement. The characteristics that Greg shares with the borderline personality reflect the pathological bereavement process in general. As has been stated, the most prominent characteristics in all pathological bereavement processes are significant ambivalence and a disturbance in selfregard, that is, anger turned inward as a result of guilt (Freud 1917; Parkes 1972).

Greg's extreme difficulties in dealing with the separation process are largely reflected in the previously described variables that are associated with the process. In the case of Greg, as with borderlines in general, the variables that affect separation are problematic and therefore are adversely influencing him in his attempt to separate from his parents during the adolescent period.

The Variables in Greg's Separation

Variable 1. The readiness of the individual for independence. In reviewing the case history, it can be seen that Greg's parents gave him the impression that he was incapable of taking care of himself. They removed the possibility for practice in the ability to take care of himself. They put him in as dependent a situation as possible and knocked down his self-esteem in any and all attempts that he made for individuation. All these put-downs gave Greg the message that he was inadequate to take care of himself, which resulted in his lack of self-esteem.

Greg made some attempts to rebel against this process. Seeing his parents either overtly or tacitly reject him when he pulled away from them, he was forced to reject them when he attempted independent functioning. He did this by running away, his way of moving toward independence. While he did a pretty poor job of taking care of himself when he ran, doing no better than living a marginal existence as a "street hustler," he did gain some sense of independence. His return home after running was more often caused by his guilt and the ambivalence associated with independence than by his marginal existence. Greg, however, sees being a "street hustler" as a poorly esteemed existence, and his self-confidence in his ability to take care of himself, based on his past experience, is correspondingly low.

During the time that I've known him, he has had greater opportunity to take care of himself in a more productive way. The halfway house has provided opportunity and support for more independent functioning. He has had opportunities that allow him to make mistakes without feeling defeated and that allow some measure of success. As a result, he has gained greater self-reliance.

Variable 2. Cognitive influences, including object constancy and the assimilative-accommodative modes of adaptation. As stated previously, the most prominent factors of cognition that affect the process of separation are the assimilation-accommodation modes of response to change and the ability to recognize patterns in object constancy and object relations. Greg's experience in interpersonal relations was chaotic and contradictory. Greg at times lacked experiences that were challenging, while at other times had experiences that were extremely anxiety-provoking. Greg therefore has not developed good assimilative and accommodative modes of response to change. He at times, will respond to change without being able to integrate its meaning into his understanding of what is happening. This is largely reflected in his "as if personality" style. When confronted with a novel situation, he will often mimic others whom he feels are successful without really understanding what is happening or the rationale for his action. That is, under stress he will exclusively accommodate to a novel situation. For instance, in the group meetings he would often act like the doctor, trying to mimic the person whom he saw as the safest one in the group.

At other times Greg deals with the anxiety of not understanding changes by fantasizing; that is, he uses an extremely assimilative mode of cognition. For example, he can see himself as a completely independent, successful musician. Although he is a good pianist, in this fantasy he completely ignores the accommodation-in this case, the tasks that are necessary for him in becoming a musician. Thus there are significant cognitive problems that keep him from effectively dealing with the separation-individuation process.

Another aspect of cognition that is causing Greg difficulty in separationindividuation is a disturbance in object constancy, or, as it has been defined, a poor ability to recognize the behavior patterns of those important to him. The excessive ambivalence that his parents felt toward him resulted in inconsistent treatment and double messages on their part.

Singer (1976) points out that in families of borderline adolescents the communication systems of action and language are incongruent. In the case of Greg this was very prevalent. The feelings that the different family members expressed by their actions toward Greg were frequently the opposite of their verbal expressions. Since children must have consistent and repetitive experiences in order to learn to understand patterns, it is clear these contradictory experiences made learning patterns extremely difficult for Greg. This difficulty in being able to recognize patterns may have something to do with Greg's and other borderline individuals' propensity to have psychotic episodes in chaotic situations. Since their cognitive ability is underdeveloped, the person in a rapidly changing situation is more likely to become confused and therefore more anxious.

The "double-bind" theory of schizophrenia (Bateson et al. 1975) is based on the communication system being contradictory. The propensity of borderline individuals for having psychotic episodes in chaotic situations can be seen in this context. A very simple example of Greg's inability to distinguish a predictable pattern was that, although the therapist came to therapy on time and missed no appointments for months, Greg did not have the cognitive understanding to predict that in the future the therapist would likely come on time. For several months, he felt surprised every time the therapist arrived. He simply was not able to extrapolate on the basis of past patterns of relationship.

Greg was very sensitive to another person's immediate mood. He could very quickly pick up subtle indications of anger, irritation, anxiety, and so forth. He based his response to the therapist on these observations, without consideration of the past experience together. In other words, Greg's ability for higher levels of abstraction in interpersonal relations lacked development; that is, he failed to recognize that a momentary mood was not as significant as an established pattern of relating. In Greg's case, this inability to recognize patterns of behavior made people less predictable and more feared. It further had an adverse effect on one of the essential components of separation identification through internalization of those aspects of people that were of value to him. Since he was not able to pick up patterns of behavior, it was very difficult for him to view a role model accurately. In other words, he often could not recognize that a person who was honest in one situation would be honest in another situation. One cannot identify with or internalize something they do not comprehend.

In treatment, the therapist's consistency was extremely important. The therapist was carefully observant of the patterns of interaction with Greg and continually verbalized them. Both verbally and nonverbally, the therapist's suggestions became predictable; therefore the therapist became predictable. Through this process Greg has become increasingly sensitive to patterns and to their predictive value. This has made his identification with his therapist and with others more accurate and thus more valuable to him. When he becomes anxious, he often feels the need to call his therapist and to reassure himself of the therapist's pattern of behavior and care for him. That the therapist has remained and has cared about him for a year still does not at times provide enough consistency for him to believe it, but there certainly has been movement in this direction.

Variable 3. The nature of the parent-child relationship. This relationship is characteristically highly ambivalent among borderline personalities on the part of both the parents and the child. Greg's relationship with his parents, for example, varied from symbiotic to rejecting. He was given some positive response for being dependent but was rejected whenever he showed any independence or individuality. He was made to feel like a bad or sick person if he acted as a separate entity. Furthermore, his mother was tremendously dependent on her children; that is, she was dependent on being needed by her family. By wanting to separate, Greg was made to feel as if he wanted to hurt his mother. This, of course, made him feel evil and guilty.

However, because of the family ambivalence about separation, he was tacitly encouraged to be separate and independent, acting out one side of their ambivalence, and then was made to feel evil for doing so, responding to the other side of their ambivalence. This was partly responsible for Greg's self-destructiveness; he would relieve his guilt for wanting to be separate and independent by punishing himself, thus feeling as though he had paid his penalty for the transgression. Self-destructiveness itself is for Greg an independent, although "sick" act and thus, on an intrapsychic level, an effective response to this ambivalence.

Variable 4. The past experiences of the parents and the adolescent in separation. Being separate and individuated within Greg's family was given a negative sanction, and the past experiences in separation were extremely troublesome. Independent desires were viewed as being very dangerous feelings to have. In essence, wanting to separate meant being rejected by the family members, especially the mother. Masterson (1972) points out that most of the parents, especially the mothers of borderlines, have borderline characteristics themselves. Their feelings are very ambivalent concerning separation and the need to be attached. Therefore, their own anxiety concerning separation is conveyed very early to their offspring. When her child begins to "separate" from her, the mother is reminded of her own feelings of abandonment, and she wants to cling. She becomes angry if the child does not respond in kind. This is especially critical during the first individuation-separation stage of development, from eighteen to thirty-six months (Mahler 1968, 1975; Masterson 1972).

Greg also got along poorly with his father. His father saw his interest in music, rather than in football or in other things that he had in his life felt proud of, as a personal rejection. Greg, on the other hand, felt that his father would accept him only if he gave up his independence, but he greatly desired his father's approval for his musical talents as a symbol of his father's true love for him as an individual. This strong ambivalence concerning independence from his father, combined with his untimely death, led to a very traumatic separation experience for Greg. It led to further anxiety and guilt associated with wanting to separate from his family.

Especially with his problems related to object constancy, Greg had, to some extent, associated his ambivalence and anger toward his father with the cause of his death. He has wondered out loud if his anger somehow caused his father to have a heart attack. Again, this makes wanting separation feel very dangerous.

Greg had the experience in his early childhood of his dog dying. He associates with this some feelings of responsibility since he mistreated the dog. He wonders if the dog went out in the middle of the street because of its mistreatment. The cognitive process here is rather undeveloped, that is, magical, in its sense of causation. Although he recognizes this rationally, the feeling of guilt remains, and it contributes to his general fear and ambivalence toward desiring separation.

As can be seen, separation in Greg's past has been an extremely painful experience; therefore there is a great urge to avoid it. Each separation reminds Greg of all previous separations.

Variable 5. The cultural influences on the separation process. In general, the cultural influences on the borderline are the same as they are on all adolescents. However, their effect on the borderline is far more pronounced. At present, the guidelines of our culture are very diverse, with the boundaries of expectation rather unclear. The adult experience is very different from the childhood experience, and the environment is quickly changing. As stated previously, one of the things that Deutsch (1942) found was that when the expectations were structured and very stable, the borderline could adequately cope in society. In other words, even though they still usually experienced depression, anxiety, and emptiness-those remained no matter what the environment-the person could, by adopting an "as if" role, maintain at least a decent adaptation to the culture. However, in an environment that is diverse and quickly changing, where the roles are rather undefined and diffuse, the borderline really has no clear-cut models and no explicit structure on which to base his role. Without this explicit structure, the borderline feels lost. In Deutsch's time, borderlines often maintained themselves well in society for long periods. Today borderlines often look to the counterculture and to religious cults to gain some explicit structure in guiding their development of "as-if" roles, and they are more apt to be accepted into these cultures.

Greg looked to the counterculture for his role mode. The counterculture also provided some support for his anger and ambivalence toward his parents. Its members had few expectations of him and accepted his sometimes bizarre behavior without looking down on him. Much of his denial of depression was given some support, and his lack of impulse control was overlooked. The counterculture did not relieve him of his feelings of anxiety, and although it gave him some opportunity to experiment with identity types, it maintained the diffusion of identity and supported it to some extent. As Greg found more self-control, more acceptance and awareness of his affect, and greater identity integration, the counterculture became less appealing.

In summary, then, Greg's developmental history has not prepared him for independence. It has created an ambivalence in his feelings toward his parents and toward himself, which has made the separation process so loaded that it is a pervasive focus of his attention at present. As can be seen from the discussion, the variables that affect the separation process were all adversely affected in his development. It is no wonder that Greg is in his present situation, having an extremely difficult time with the bereavement process.

The Stages in Greg's Separation

The analogy, discussed in Chapter 7, relating the learning of skiing to an adolescent progressing through the stages of separation aptly applies to Greg's progression through the stages as well. That is, he progressed only after alternating progressive and regressive movement.

When the therapist first met Greg, he was dealing primarily with the issues of the first stages of the bereavement process. The mountains in his past had been too steep and had resulted in many falls, making him lose confidence in proceeding further. Also, he did not have a good model or teacher to help him learn how to get down the hill. At times he tried to get down the mountain as fast as possible using the most advanced technique-for example, running away before he really felt independent. The result was more bad spills.

Greg has begun to deal with issues of the separation process more realistically. As a result, he is beginning to move through the stages. When situations became tough, though, like the skier on a too-steep mountain, he regresses. He also tries to move too quickly at times, causing a spill and, again, regression. On the whole, however, Greg is moving toward greater individuation-separation at present.

Stage 1. Control of impulse to reattach. In the beginning of therapy, Greg often had periods of fear of losing control, of becoming enraged, or of wanting to run home to his mother or father, although he was very aware that his father was not there. He was angered and frightened by these impulses. There was a great deal of identity diffusion. At times he felt like the child of his parents, and at other times like a separated adult. All of these things will be recognized as issues of the first stage of separation. Greg, for the most part, denied and acted out these feelings rather than really coming to terms with them. When he first began therapy, he often had feelings of wanting to be attached to his mother, and his urge to return to her was so strong that he felt he would have to destroy her in order to destroy the feeling. Similar feeling toward his father ultimately led to his tremendous guilt toward his father's death. He also, in these early stages, would direct analogous feelings toward the therapist, being enraged at the limits of the relationship, wanting to establish a symbiotic relationship, and trying to get as much attention as possible-in essence not allowing the therapist any room to be himself. At other times, he rejected all feelings of closeness to the therapist.

During the past year, Greg has lived in secure and structured environments. He has been in psychotherapy consistently. In this context, the consistency of the therapeutic attachment has been repeatedly pointed out, while at the same time, the limits of the relationship have been verbalized. The halfway house and the therapist have both supported, and at times enforced, limits on acting out behavior. The therapist has, at the same time, related this acting out behavior to the impulse to reattach. Over the past year, Greg has learned more and more to face these feelings and to gain understanding and control over them. Hence there has been at least a partial resolution of Stage 1.

Stage 2. The cognitive realization of the separation. At first in therapy, Greg largely acted out these issues impulsively. His running away and selfdestructive behaviors were, at least in part, aimed at proving his independence from his parents. He also took on counterculture belief systems in opposition to his parents' views, again aimed at demonstrating his separateness.

At this point, any suggestion that Greg shared a similar point of view with his parents was seen as tantamount to saying that he still had a childlike attachment to them. He also had periodic fears of being separate. At these times he would disavow his counterculture beliefs and engage in activities he felt would please his parents. His attempt at working for his brother was one such period.

The overriding issue, however, remained separation, and soon he would become angry at himself for his dependency. He often despaired during these periods that things were going nowhere. Again, the impulsive reactions to the dependent feeling would return, and correspondingly the behaviors aimed at proving separation-the counterculture belief systems, panhandling, dope dealing, and self-destructive behavior-returned.

In therapy genuinely self-reliant and self-supporting behavior has been strongly encouraged and reinforced. Greg has taken some steps in becoming more self-reliant. In the halfway house where he lives he has taken on greater responsibility than is required. For example, along with the requirements of helping to cook meals, he has also been house manager. He has become very frugal in managing his own money. He has taken on the responsibility for dealing with the welfare department entirely without assistance. He has also taken some steps to get enrolled in college, with the ultimate goal of being a piano teacher. These successful independent activities have given Greg some sense that he is capable of independence and that he has made movement in these areas.

There has been, in the course of therapy, occasion for both agreement and disagreement on questions of the day, such as politics, cultural norms, and aesthetics. Care was taken in pointing out after these discussions that Greg was respected and cared for whether he agreed with the therapist or not and that disagreement was not rejection. On a number of occasions, it has been suggested that Greg and his mother had used political arguments as symbols of their discord over separation. Greg would state how different his views were from his mother's, and she would say how bad he was for having those views.

Greg has become less counterculture-oriented recently. However, he still often goes into long put-downs of his parents' "conventional" views.

Greg has made considerable gains in viewing himself independently from his parents. He has had very little contact with his mother lately, and although he feels good about seeing himself grow more independent, he also feels bad that his mother will not see him. When these feelings become particularly intense, he again sees himself as being dependent and regresses somewhat. On the whole, however, he has gained a new confidence that he can live without her. He has also become more relieved that his separation is not leading to his mother's destruction. Sometimes he has dreams in which he has caused her death, but he has come to believe his independence will not destroy his mother and that he is, therefore, not evil in wanting to separate. Again, these feelings are not fully stable, but there is on the whole an acknowledgment and commitment to his being on the road to independence, signaling a partial resolution of the issues of Stage 2.

Stage 3. The affective response to the separation. The issues of this stage are those that are presently most central to Greg. He is continually battling feelings associated with the ever-growing realization of his separationfeelings of loneliness and isolation and associated feelings of guilt related to his responsibility for the attenuation of the relationship. Greg is searching for a new meaning and value in his pursuit of a more independent relationship with his parents. (This is, for the most part, taking place within himself.) This is what Parkes referred to as "mitigation of the separation." As a result of these issues, Greg is experiencing frequent depressive periods, along with withdrawn loneliness. He has often stated during these periods that he feels as though something is dying.

During these periods he often isolates himself and despairs that the depression will never end. At times he also is troubled by dreams of death, often with either him or his mother as the victim. He suffers sleepless nights as a result. He is also troubled during these periods with suicidal ideation.

These suicidal feelings can be related to Alvarez's discussion of suicide in *The Savage God* (1971). He states that suicidal feelings are a message that something within the person is so painful it must die. The battle, as Alvarez sees it, it to separate the part that must die from the rest of the individual. This is the case with Greg. If he can allow his childhood relationship with his parents to die, the adult in him will be free to live. As can be seen, this is a painful battle. When Greg confronted these feelings initially, he tended to regress to earlier stages and tried to avoid facing them. He employed all of the defense mechanisms discussed previously.

The therapist attempted to give meaning to the depression. Greg was told in essence that by facing the loneliness he would gain a sense of independence that would ultimately give him a sense of accomplishment and, by doing so, dispel the depression. By giving up his dependency, he would open himself up to new kinds of relationships, leading him out of the loneliness.

The therapist does not play down the depression nor helps Greg to avoid it. It is obviously a miserable experience for Greg to face. An attempt is made to support Greg's successful handling of the depression by giving him well-deserved praise for facing a tough battle. He is especially supported when his feeling of depression is related to his gaining some independence of the therapist; this opportunity is used to confront the guilt he associates with becoming independent. On occasion Greg has asked how the therapist would feel if he was not needed anymore. He was told that the therapist must also be willing to give something up if he is to get something in return. The therapist must give up Greg's dependency on him if he is to enjoy the feeling that they have accomplished something together.

Greg has become more able to face his feelings of depression without regressive behavior. He can better confront the feeling of despair that the depressions will never end. He has been rewarded for his perseverance by seeing that after a period of time, the depressive periods do attenuate; he has thus gained a sense of accomplishment and more confidence in his ability to face them. At times he returns to his previous ways of dealing with the depression, but he is doing this less and less.

Greg is now most focused on the issues of Stage 3. He is battling to feel good about his separateness, to feel an openness to new relationships rather than depression. The battle is far from over, but it is progressing.

Stage 4. Identification. The issue of this stage, identification with the separated person, is not as yet a central concern for Greg in relationship to his parents, since he has not yet resolved the issues of Stage 3. Unfortunately, this stage will be no less difficult than the other stages. Even when Greg feels more comfortable in his separateness from his parents, identification with them will be problematic because the ambivalence and guilt will likely never be fully resolved. For this to happen with his mother she would have to be willing to give him permission and her blessings for being a separate, different individual-a very unlikely occurrence. Up to this point she has continually rejected him.

The identification can, therefore, only take place with the ambivalence and guilt remaining as factors. Identification with one who rejects may take place only by internalizing the rejection as well.

What can be hoped for is that Greg, through gaining a greater understanding of his mother and a greater acceptance of himself, will gain some resolution of the ambivalence and guilt he feels toward his mother. Possibly, if he learns how to forgive himself, he will be able to forgive his parents, and vice versa. He will thereby open up the possibility of accepting the ways in which he is like his parents, of seeing what parts of the relationship were rewarding to him, and of internalizing those. In so doing, he can identify with them less ambivalently and thus more fully accept himself. It is more realistic to foresee this issue as remaining to some extent problematic.

He may be able to resolve this loss partially by substituting parental figures, such as the therapist, with whom he can identify. In therapy, an attempt has been made to allow him to feel good about this identification. On many occasions his feelings of wanting to be like the therapist have been discussed. For example, Greg has talked about entering the mental health field by doing music therapy. He has wondered out loud if the therapist had objections to this ambition. On many occasions he has pointed out times when he helped others through difficult periods, stating that he had done as well as his therapist could have. He has professed to others the importance of the main goal in therapy—openness and honesty within a relationship. He is thereby using the therapist as a parental role model with whom he can identify. As he has stated, "You are more of a father to me than my real father."

Stage 5. The attenuation of the child-parent relationship and the corresponding development of a new relationship. This stage is still unentered territory for Greg. He has begun to talk about the goal of independence from his parents and his therapist. Much of this is on a fantasy level at present. He has talked of what it would be like to be friends with his mother. He has also wondered what it would be like if he no longer came to therapy. He has asked if he could still be friends with the therapist if he was no longer a patient. As stated in the case history, he discussed seeing another therapist because he wanted the opportunity to explore a more adult-to-adult relationship, one in which he is not as dependent as he is in his current relationship. He recognizes that he sees his therapist doing many of the things that a parent would do for him interpersonally. He is ambivalent toward these now, as he is ambivalent toward being a child; this ambivalence is part of his drive to be separate.

It has been pointed out that Greg can continue to see his therapist but with a changed relationship, with his being less dependent on him. This is a goal that both can work toward. The door has also been left open for him to see somebody else if he wants to in the future. He states that he has no desire to terminate at this time but sees this as a goal for the future. He has also begun to talk about what it will be like being on his own. At present, however, these are only seen as goals for the future.

The Treatment Strategy

In conclusion, the variables of the separation process have, in Greg's case, all been experienced negatively. As a result, Greg has been pathologically stuck in an ambivalent relationship with his mother and deceased father. The therapeutic response has been to enter into a relationship with Greg that initially reflected a child-parent relationship and that moved toward a more adult-to-adult relationship. The experience of this relationship has been therapeutic by providing a good experience working through the stages of separation. This, then, provides a basis for working through the separation from Greg's parents. Masterson (1972, 1976), who has worked extensively with borderline patients, bases his treatment program on helping the individual work through the bereavement for the lost mother figure.

The discussion of Greg's treatment not only is valuable for the treatment of borderline patients but has further implications for helping individuals with less severe struggles related to adolescent-parental separation. Pfeiffer (1974, p. 218) has noted this relationship between the borderline struggle and the adolescent struggle:

> The reader may have noticed already that to a certain extent the suggested approach to the borderline patient is similar to that used with adolescents. That is intended. Adolescents and borderline patients both face somewhat similar tasks, integration of new experiences, expanding complexity of interactions, identity formation of solidification. It is therefore not merely coincidental that similar approaches can be employed and, not incidentally, often with similarly good results. Both are growth situations.

Part IV
OVERCOMING PROBLEMS OF THE
SEPARATION PROCESS

CHAPTER 13

Psychotherapy and Other Developmental Experiences

The process of adolescent-parental separation is at times troublesome. Most parents and teenagers can take this in stride. However, for some it is experienced as quite painful and can lead to long-term problems. In others—for example, the borderline adolescent—it is experienced as intolerable much of the time. Some who feel overburdened by problems during this period seek help from mental health professionals or others. What follows in this chapter is a discussion of some of the experiences and interactions that appear helpful to parents and teenagers burdened by the adolescent-parental separation process.

Intervention in Nonpathological Cases of Separation

Many parents and teenagers who are troubled by the process are, in fact, moving toward separation quite well. Frequently these people, however, seek counseling because they believe something is wrong. Most frequently this consists of the parents regarding their teenagers as being rebellious in a way quite different from that of their own adolescent period. Without the background to understand this, parents are often worried that their teenagers' rebellion means the beginnings of an antisocial pattern that will culminate in their teenagers' becoming permanently alienated from the culture and from them. Parents may fear that their teenager is becoming a criminal. Further, they are quite troubled by the teenager's rebellion because they experience it as a form of permanent rejection, feeling as though they somehow failed as parents. In such cases, educating the family members to the process of separation and redefining the events as nonpathological can be quite effective intervention. The following case illustrates such a family.

The parents of a fourteen-year-old boy seek counseling for him, who is their eldest son, because in their words, "He has begun behaving quite different of late." He no longer wanted to do anything with the family, frequently got into arguments with them, and at times came home after curfew. His grades had dropped from primarily As to Cs and Bs, and on three occasions over the past three months he had come in after going drinking with some friends. The parents felt that these friends were not on a "par" with their teenage boy. The teenager felt that his parents were overprotective of him. He felt he should have later hours; he did not think that his coming in after drinking on several occasions was any "big deal"; and he stated that his grades at school were improving but that he had dropped mainly because he did not like several of his teachers. In short, the issues that the family were describing were primarily the issues discussed previously as being within the boundaries of the common adolescent-parental separation process.

After listening to the teenager as well as the parents, the issues surrounding the process of separation, including the role of rebellion and the testing of limits as proving and finding one's individuality, were discussed with everyone. Within this context the importance of the parents' maintaining their integrity and their belief system as well as providing consistent limits where necessary was stressed. There was an obvious sigh of relief by all concerned. A follow-up meeting was held approximately a month later, and all members of the family agreed that, in fact, little had changed but that everybody felt better. This family stated that six months later all was still going well.

This case illustrates the value of education, or, as the communication theorists would call it, *reframing* (Watzlawick 1978). That is, when these people first came in they saw each others' behavior as rejecting, destructive, and angry. When they left, the same behavior was seen as a developmental process, thus bringing a great relief to all concerned.

Other people who are troubled by the separation process may need more intensive intervention when the process has become stuck or unduly painful and/or causes behavior that is destructive in both the short-run and the long-run. Some of these people's attempts to resolve the adolescentparental separation process leads only to greater pain, despair, and entrenchment in the pattern. If these people are to work through the separation process, some change must occur within the individual or the social system to allow for further resolution and development.

It is perplexing that people can suffer significantly, have good insight into what causes their suffering, and yet not change. In situations where there is obvious abuse, repression, or deprivation, people frequently can see the enemy and plot the strategy for escape, especially teenagers. Other people who on the surface look like they should be happy still suffer and, it appears, work hard at creating their own suffering. Consider the following example.

Two married people appear to others, and possibly to themselves, to be happy. They rarely argue and get along well with their children. Their oldest boy reaches adolescence. The husband steps out on his wife, making it obvious enough for her to catch him. Soon they are both suffering over the loss of their relationship. Whether they remain living together or not, they feel separated. The suffering may lead to the terrible pain of depression. People may suggest changes to them. They may see alternatives that are hopeful, yet they do not change.

People sometimes hurt those they love. Sometimes they are unaware of the pain they are causing, and other times they are aware. They may wish to stop the suffering. They may be motivated to change and may try to change, yet change does not occur. Usually they see the suffering, but they do not see they avoid at all cost seeing the suffering as a result of their own behavior. They explain the behavior as being caused by other people or by circumstances. In describing Milton Erikson's process of "weaning parents from children" Haley (1973) points out, for example, that it is the loving parent who is attempting to make life as pleasurable as possible for his or her teenager while maintaining an overly involved relationship who ultimately causes the most difficulties for the teenager during this period. If the parents were less loving, the teenager's escape would be easier, for he or she would be able to reject the parents' behavior with less ambivalence and guilt.

A mother and father come to a therapist and say that their daughter is getting into trouble. They meet with the therapist several times and discover together that the daughter is overly rebellious because she is being smothered by parental love. The parents resolve to do things differently. The next week they are unable to make the meeting. During the following weeks they miss every appointment and state that they do not have the time to come in anymore, but that things are no better. The parents are trying to stop the suffering caused by their daughter's increasing independence. This brings them into therapy. The daughter came into therapy to relieve the suffering caused by the guilt resulting from her parents' reaction to her move toward greater independence. This was largely unconscious. When the involvement in therapy means uncovering the cause of the pain, all are involved. When the issue becomes change, all members begin to withdraw.

When people suffer significantly from a loss or an anticipated loss, they frequently seek help from friends, clergy, and psychotherapists. When support or education suffices to relieve pain and to allow the individual to proceed through the separation process, the person is open to the help, as in the first case presented here. However, if the pain continues and it becomes apparent that the individual or the individual's family must change in order for the process to progress, the issues become much more problematic since change appears even more uncomfortable than the suffering. What makes change so difficult that people would resist it even at the expense of maintaining their suffering? The following discussion of this question is not meant as a comprehensive answer but as one that has been found to be helpful in aiding people to change.

Resistance to Change

Consistency and stability are important to all of us. Every day we have numerous interactions with people in which we know with relative comfort what their response will be to our action, therefore we give it little conscious thought. If we change our way of doing things, we must first give up this accepted reciprocity. That is, if we do something different or unusual, we can expect the response to be different and unusual. Ethologists as well as psychologists have discussed at length the value and the power of habit. Fear of the unknown is common to all of us and must be resolved so that change may occur. One becomes acutely aware of the value of reciprocal expectations when one changes jobs, schools, or neighborhoods. He or she becomes very anxious in dealing with these new situations; life becomes less predictable and therefore far more of a challenge with the anxiety of the unknown. If the changes are significant enough, our very sense of self, that is, our identity, becomes unknown to us. We do not know how we will now respond in old situations given our new outlook and the changes that we have made in ourselves; therefore, old situations become new situations, and we become unknown even to ourselves. When we change, we suffer a certain loss of meaning until we are able to find continuity between what we have valued in the past and what we are doing in the present.

Even in deciding on a course of change, one suffers a loss of self-esteem. That is, the decision to make a change entails accepting to some extent that what one did in the past was not good enough, that somehow, in some way, one has failed. If this involves an interpersonal relationship, then the decision to make a change may even mean accepting that in some ways we have done harm to somebody else-we may feel a sense of guilt if we accept the need to change. Therefore, change may be avoided quite strenuously to avoid this guilt.

There is another danger to self-esteem. As long as we keep doing things the way in which we have always done them, even if we admit to ourselves that we need to change, we avoid failing at change. If we try to change, we may fail in our endeavors. Thus we risk a new failure, another affront to our self-esteem.

Another resistance to change involves the needs of the social network, which, like the individual, is most comfortable with the past predictable outcomes that are presently being drawn from the group for use in maintaining the satisfaction of needs. The family is usually the most important social system in this regard. A change in an individual in the family can cause other members to have to change their expectations and satisfactions as well.

Take the case of Dolly, sixteen years old, who for years has talked of dieting. She and her mother are the overweight members of the family, and they are overly dependent on one another. Dolly is the child aligned with the mother, while the other children align themselves with their father. Food is the mechanism through which the mother shares love with Dolly, making eating a part of accepting love. To diet may mean to reject the mother's love. The other siblings see fat Dolly as nonthreatening, since their self-esteem has come from being athletic, good-looking children, taking after their father. Thus a change in body image may force a change in competitiveness as well. Her obesity serves a number of functions in this regard—for example, it inhibits her relations with boys, thus inhibiting her moving away from her mother in the context of a heterosexual relationship. While overtly the overweight girl may get encouragement for reducing, she also picks up the message that staying the same would make her family rest easier.

Although this discussion of resistances to change is far from complete, one can see that while change may rationally be desirable, there is a great deal that one must confront in order for change to occur. Further, most of this resistance is unconscious.

The patterns of interaction, then, that maintain parent-adolescent interdependence must undergo a change which, like all changes, is resisted. For the adolescent to move toward independence, this resistance must be confronted successfully as well as the problems directly affecting the separation process. This is indeed a formidable task.

In a sense, this discussion of change to allow separation is circular in that change is in itself a separation from what one has done and has been in the past. One must again give something up to get something new. Thus the variables that affect separation are also prominent forces in change itself. In the case of adolescent-parental separation, the coalescence of biological and cultural impetuses powerfully motivates adolescents and parents to confront the resistance to change despite the pain. It is the therapist's goal to direct this motivation in such a way that change can be best accepted while the separation constructively takes place. Following is a summary of the therapeutic interventions that have been found to be most useful.

Useful Therapeutic Interventions

The most common dynamic that causes problems in the separation process is parents who are not able to deal with the loss of the fulfillment of needs that was provided by the child and who, as a result, either verbally or nonverbally communicate this to the teenager, causing the teenager to feel guilty. In terms of the variables that have been discussed, the most prominent influence is the parents' lack of readiness for the separation process and the corresponding quality of the parent-child relationship, which is filled with ambivalence. As Haley (1976) points out, this frequently entails a parent who is overly involved with the teenager, to the exclusion of the other parent.

In his book, *Uncommon Therapy* (1973), Haley describes Milton Erickson's therapeutic process of "weaning parents from children." As Haley describes it, Erickson sees this therapy as a process where the parents and teenagers experience each other as disengaged from each other and then reengage in a new way. This is reminiscent of the initiation rites that were discussed in Chapter 5-initiation rites being an experience where the parents see the teenager as separate and then as a fellow adult. The initiation rite, as was stated, reflects in an analogous way the process of separation. Erickson uses his innovative understanding of hypnotic suggestion (not necessarily in a trance state) to develop his own initiation rites. He does this in two stages. The initial phase is separating the parent and the teenager so that they experience each other as more independent. Erickson tries to develop a situation where the teenager must operate more independently and the parents must observe this greater autonomy. He then seeks to create a situation where an individual's needs are better satisfied by a more autonomous relationship of parents and child. For example, he may set up a situation, while the teenager is outside the home, in which the parents may experience their closeness to each other in a new way, thus relieving the teenager of providing for this closeness.

Family Therapy

In my work with parents and teenagers, I have found family therapy to be most expedient for creating experiences leading to growing separation between parents and teenagers. This appears most effective because first, the problems are usually interactional ones that do not originate solely in one individual and that therefore are difficult for one individual to alter. Second, the resistances to change are to some extent circumvented in family therapy. Changes that one must make are set forth primarily in relationship to other family members. Therefore, the individual's identity is not seen as altering in such a significant way as when someone goes into individual therapy, wanting to change. Further, problems can be set forth as habits of interacting with one another, therefore avoiding the placing of responsibility on any one individual, which would result in loss of self-esteem. Finally, the family members may be less fearful of failing at change, since responsibility is shared.

One must, however, deal with guilt on a family interactional level. Family members, to avoid their own guilt for things that have gone badly in the past, often attempt to put the blame or the responsibility on other members of the family. Since everyone in the family wishes to avoid guilt, this tends to inhibit the willingness to accept responsibility for change. Another problem often centers around family members' protecting each other from blame, that is, guilt. Blame may be avoided, however, if past problems are put in terms of interactional habits that must be altered moving the focus away from blame and guilt and therefore allowing the family members to change without feeling as though they had been harmful to other members in the past. Alternatively, the therapist can show them that the protecting of others in the family is an act of love. This reframes the meaning of the activity, from weakness to love. Change can occur much more readily with this positive understanding.

The following case presents an example of a family experiencing difficulty in the separation process and developing new interactional patterns, which allows them to become more independent in a way that is more satisfying for all family members.

Claire's Case. Claire, a fifteen-year-old girl, was admitted to an adolescent treatment program after she had taken an overdose of drugs. This was her second suicide attempt in a three-month period. She had also run away from home on three occasions and had been a drug abuser for a year. She stated that she had taken the overdose because she had been ostracized by her friends recently. After talking to her parents and with her further, it became apparent that Claire had run away and had attempted suicide after getting into arguments with her parents and feeling rejected. These arguments had become increasingly more painful to both her and her parents over a period of about a year. Prior to that they had had a good relationship. Claire was the oldest of four children; she was close to her next younger sister, who was two years her junior, and was somewhat distant from her brother, who was four years younger, and from her sister, who was five years younger. The other children in the family got along very well with the parents, although the sister close to Claire felt that the parents sometimes picked on Claire.

The initial meetings with the family, which extended over a two-week period, dealt primarily with each family member's being given opportunities to discuss how they saw the issues related to Claire's problems. Initially Claire was very reluctant to talk in front of her parents, fearing that their feelings would be hurt and that they would retaliate. However, during the two-week period she became increasingly comfortable in discussing her views openly. The parents also initially were defensive, fearing that they would be blamed for what had happened. However, when blame was clearly kept out of the discussion, the parents more comfortably gave views on what they felt was going on. The parents' view of the problem was that Claire had generally been a good girl until about a year prior to her running away and attempting suicide. They stated that she had become friends with a boy and a girl who had influenced her to get involved with drugs and to rebel against her parents. Claire's view of the situation was that her parents were overly controlling of her and that they picked on her.

During the year prior to Claire's admission to the adolescent program, her parents, as they stated, had been very child-centered. Most of their activities together had been focused on the children. They had had their children soon after they were married. As a result, their way of being close was always having the children as their center of focus. Approximately a year before Claire's admittance, Claire's friends had become increasingly more important to her, and she began to feel like doing things more with her friends than with her family, a natural move toward independence for a fourteen-year-old. The younger sister, who was twelve, followed Claire's lead and also began to feel like doing things that were less involved with the family. The parents found themselves having less contact with their children and thus felt threatened with having less contact with each other. They began to feel themselves as being denied intimacy, and they reacted by becoming angry.

Their initial arguments were directed toward each other. The arguments became heated; on at least one occasion the mother left for most of the night. She never told the children or the father where she had gone. It was several weeks after this event that Claire first ran away. The parents then became involved with the police department and their family doctor regarding the runaway. This brought them closer together. About a month later the parents again began to argue, and it was about a week after that that Claire got into a fight with her parents and made her first suicide attempt. This cycle continued for the next several months, until Claire was brought into the adolescent program.

In assessing the situation, one can see that Claire was caught between her own motivation for independence and separation and her parents' needs. The message that she received from her parents through their actions was that her independence left their needs unsatisfied. This left Claire in a position of feeling guilty and ambivalent about her own feelings of separation. Her resolution was to act out in such a way that it brought her parents together around her, the problem child. This was, of course, largely unconscious.

The goals of treatment were to prepare the parents for Claire's separation in a way that was nondestructive, while at the same time getting the message to Claire that separation was acceptable, relieving her of the guilt. It was felt that an interpretation of this would probably not be understood fully, would make the individual involved feel guilty, and would therefore be of little value to the change process. Instead, situations were to be created that would bring the parents closer together while allowing Claire to disengage. Initially this was done during therapy, and then it was allowed gradually to take place outside of the therapeutic treatment setting.

First prescribed for the parents was the task of developing a set of appropriate limits for Claire. They had some major disagreement regarding this, the mother being more lenient than the father. With the focus remaining on agreeing on limits for Claire, attention was paid to the difficulties the parents had in solving their conflict. At several points Claire attempted to get into arguments with her parents in order to rescue them from arguing with each other. Initially, the therapist stopped Claire's interventions. Later, the parents began doing so themselves.

In working with the parents on these differences, it was apparent that conflict resolution in general was a problem. Their attempts to resolve their differences usually ended up making them frustrated, angry, and feeling more distant. A meeting was held at this point without Claire, again focusing on the parents' resolving their differences around discipline. In this setting they were able to come to some agreements. It was obvious that as a result they felt much closer to one another.

To enhance this closeness, it was suggested that they would probably complete the plan for Claire if they spent a weekend away from the children. They had not taken a vacation away from their children in years. The parents needed little encouragement for this at this point. The next weekend the parents made arrangements with the grandmother, who lived close by, to take care of the children while they went off for a weekend together to develop this treatment plan. In the following session, the parents presented the plan as a united front. Claire tested out the plan by aligning herself with her mother on one point, attempting to get her mother and father into conflict. However, her mother and father remained united in their presentation of the limits that Claire would be expected to follow. The parents further let it be known in this meeting that they had had a good time together. Claire was obviously relieved.

The following weekend Claire was home for three days. During this period of time, she tested some of the limits, coming in late on one occasion. As a result, she was given the punishment of not being allowed to go out the next night. She accepted this well, without any of the tantrums or threats to run away or to harm herself as had been heard in the past.

During the following week, Claire, in an individual meeting with her therapist, brought up her feelings of fear that her parents were headed for a divorce. The timing of her bringing this up makes it evident that she was no longer so afraid. With her therapist's encouragement, she later in the week brought this up to her parents. Her parents related that they had been having a difficult time and had had thoughts of divorce but that they felt that that time had now passed. It was evident that the parents did feel more comfortable about their involvement with each other without the children being needed so much as a catalyst. Claire was then discharged from the program.

In a follow-up meeting approximately a month and a half later, all was going well. Claire had occasionally broken rules, but she had accepted the punishment. The parents felt that they were getting along much better with each other and with the children as well. In a telephone conversation about six months later with the referring doctor, things were said to be still going very well. In some respects, however, this family especially the parents, made shifts in the relationship more rapidly than is typical. The interventions involved in this case generally represent the most useful tools in promoting healthy separation.

Individual Psychotherapy In some situations, an individual who is experiencing problems related to separation from parents will seek therapy, but family therapy will not be possible or optimum. Circumstances have occurred, for example, when the parents feel little discomfort in the situation and therefore have little motivation for the painful process of change. Family therapy may not be possible or optimum when the parents and the grown offspring live far apart or when the parents have no faith that change can occur. In some situations, a way can be found to involve parents at some point in the process. At other times, the person must be dealt with individually. I have had little success in working with adolescents who still live with their parents unless the parents are involved. However, this is not the case for young adults who have moved away from home. Individual therapy can be quite helpful with people experiencing problems in separation who are living outside their home. The lack of parental involvement does not necessarily mean defeat, especially since those who achieve separation from parents in individual therapy frequently experience an uplift in self-esteem for their accomplishment, which they may not have had in family therapy.

In the case of Greg Davis, which was discussed in Chapter 12, it would have been very helpful if Greg's mother would have been involved in therapy. However, because of distance, and more important, because of her passive avoidance of therapy, her involvement was not possible. His father, as stated, had died. Despite the noninvolvement of the parents in his therapy, Greg still experienced significant changes. Therapy was oriented toward helping him work through issues of separation first directed at the therapist, which he then transferred to his relations with others, especially his parents. The more traditional goals of psychotherapy, such as insight and the interpretation of process, were of ancillary importance. That is, at times they were focused upon, but only insofar as they expedited the process of the growing independence of Greg from the therapist.

The Therapeutic Relationship as a Model

The use of the therapeutic relationship as a model experience is valuable and important in helping people involved in disturbed separation processes that are much less pathological than the borderline syndrome. The use of the therapeutic relationship as a model is certainly not new to the field. Freud's discussion of the role of transference first brought this to light. Sullivan (1940, 1953) made an impact on psychotherapy in pointing out the primary importance of this relationship as a model, which put even more emphasis on the relationship. Sullivan's work emphasized the model as primarily overcoming issues of inability to form attachment rather than issues of separation. Rank (1945) and Kaiser (1965) focused directly on the therapeutic experience as being a model process of separation. Rank puts this in terms of the battle of will and guilt, will being the motivation to be a separate individual, and guilt being the major block that inhibits the individual from separating from parents. He states (1945, p. 101):

> This whole development from neurotic consciousness of guilt as consequence of will conflict, and its denial to the reactive guilt of differing experience culminates in the last phase of the therapeutic process and is brought to release and solution through the setting of an ending which is suitable for the particular person, both as to time and meaning. Certainly this is not the individual's first attempt to free himself, but is one which should succeed. It can only succeed, however, if one lets him accomplish himself so that he has no debt of gratitude to pay. However, this is possible in the actual therapeutic experience and not historically, no matter whether the individual feels gratitude towards his parents (and other objects) or not.

Both Kaiser and Rank start out the therapeutic process by working to form an attachment. However, when the attachment is formed, the focus shifts toward helping the individual work toward an ever-increasing individuality.

In the therapeutic process, I pay a great deal of attention to the communication system-both verbal and nonverbal-that is established and attempt to be as sensitive as possible to any contradictory messages related to dependence and independence. If any contradictions are noted, an attempt is made to assess where they are coming from. Are they a result of my feelings toward this individual's dependence on me? Are they a result of the patients feelings toward me? What is in the way of the patient's moving toward separation, and how might this be resolved? In a sense, I see myself as an exemplary parent who is helping the individual to not need me anymore.

This

is frequently a struggle not only for the patient but also for the therapist. Therapists, just as parents, need to be needed. They go into training as psychotherapists because they want to be helpful and useful to people; in a sense, though, good therapy is making yourself useless to someone, a task that is very difficult for many.

This can be seen more clearly in a very simple example of the therapeutic process. In certain forms of psychotherapy, making a good interpretation is the epitome of being a good therapist. However, I see this as a contradiction. It may make a therapist feel very good if he or she interprets an individual's behavior in what is seen as a most brilliant manner. However, in many cases this therapeutic interpretation may have a derogatory effect on the therapeutic outcome, for it may make patients feel as though they could never have provided that interpretation for themselves and that therefore, in order to straighten themselves out, they must depend on the psychotherapist. So, although the "brilliant" interpretation may make the therapist feel awfully brilliant, it is not helpful to the patient. When, however, an opportunity is provided for patients to make such interpretations for themselves, they are, in effect, finding that they no longer need the therapist. This is also true of other interactions, such as the decision-making processes.

Patients frequently ask advice, and therapists frequently give it. Certain situations may mandate this, but it usually promotes dependency. Even if the advice is highly useful, the message is clearly the therapist stating, "I make better decisions than you do," that is, "You need me."

One aspect of therapy involves a constant struggle for the therapist. In order to accomplish what is hoped will be accomplished, the therapist must fight against needs within himself, for example, need to be looked up to by the patient rather than to be ultimately seen on a horizontal plane with him. In a sense, when the therapist has done the best job, the individual will say on termination, "I've changed a lot; I feel I've accomplished what I set out to accomplish. I probably could have done it without you." What a feeling of independence this individual has felt! Implicit in this, and in order for this to occur, the therapist must, of course, start out with an attitude of respect for the patient's abilities to ultimately provide for himself or herself.

The therapeutic process, when used in helping separation to occur, then, is a model that gives the individual an experience in moving from a dependent relationship to one that is independent. The success of this process is based on the ability of the therapist to promote this movement without the relationship becoming stuck, as did the one with the parents. Therapists must do what good parents do, that is, give individuals the message that they are able to take care of themselves, without giving them the message of rejection. As in working with borderline patients, variables that inhibit the movement toward separation must be directly confronted. For example, the person may need to be directed to have experiences leading to a greater sense of financial independence. Activities to promote peer relations may be helpful if this variable has been negatively influenced. One may question this direction, seeing it as a contradiction to the person's learning independence. The rejoinder to this can be found by looking at the healthy parent-adolescent separation process. In the initial stages the parents are still very involved in directing the young teenager toward activities that will make him or her feel confident in the ability to be independent. In a similar way in the initial stages of therapy, the therapist may find it useful to direct the patient to have experiences that will make him or her more confident to be independent. The movement and expectation must be, however, toward the patient's providing this motivation for himself or herself. In the final stages of therapy this type of direction would be counterproductive, since the therapist would expect individuals to be doing this for themselves.

In conclusion, the process of conducting psychotherapy with individuals experiencing problems in separation is a process of providing a corrective experience, that is, giving them experiences of feeling good about being grown-up, separate individuals where they have been fearful or guilty about this because of past experiences. It is useful to have some awareness of what has gone awry with the separation in the past, not because this insight will create change, but because it may be helpful to the therapist in providing corrective experiences. Above all, the therapist should be the model parental figure, helping to move the relationship with the patient from a dependent one to a more symmetrical one.

In many cases, the lack of resolution of the parental-adolescent separation process carries through into later life, even to old age. For example, in my practice, there have been cases where people have been involved in repeated divorces-upon forming a relationship, they would become rebellious, treating their spouse just as they would a parent, rebelling against them, seeing them as overcontrolling, and upon becoming married, immediately beginning to work toward becoming more separate. Upon separation they would still feel unresolved, as they had not, in fact, truly dealt with the conflicts revolving around the adolescent-parental separation; hence they repeat the experience later with a new spouse.

Another example of this is parents who, because of their own ambivalence toward separating from their parents, become overly clinging toward their own children.

The following case will provide an example of how a therapeutic relationship can serve as a model to help the individual stuck in an overly dependent relationship with parents find greater independence and therefore more freedom in life pursuits. In following the therapeutic process, it will be valuable to focus some attention on how each successive stage of separation in the patient was first directed toward separating from the therapist, which in turn served as a model for the patient's separation from her mother.

Lana's Case. A twenty-nine-year-old woman came in to psychotherapy because she felt a lack of direction; she had difficulty forming satisfying relationships with men, and she was generally dissatisfied with her life. She had been married for several years and had a young child, and yet she had never lived more than a few blocks away from her mother. It soon became evident that her lack of direction and difficulties with men was related to her inability to detach herself from her relationship with her mother.

When Lana first came to see me she had been divorced 2 ½ years and had a 2 ½-year-old child from her only marriage. Lana had worked for approximately four years as a teacher, the last two as a special education teacher. She evidently did well at her job. She was a bright, insightful woman, and she talked comfortably. She lived in the San Francisco Bay area in California, where she had grown up.

Lana was an only child. Her mother and father had met when her father was in the service during World War II. Her father and mother spent little time with each other. The courtship was a short one, and the father was soon off to the war. Following the war, they lived together for a brief period of time and then were divorced. Lana and her mother then moved in with her grandmother, and shortly following that, her aunt and her aunt's two daughters moved into the house. The house was composed totally of women and girls. Lana, throughout her development, had little male contact. The grandmother was the matriarch of the household. It was her house, and she maintained control over it.

Lana's mother went to work, as did her aunt, and the grandmother took care of the house and made the meals. As there were not enough jobs to go around for the women, the children had no responsibility within the household and thus little opportunity to learn responsibility. Lana said that there was constant tension between her mother and her aunt, which got so bad when Lana was in high school that she and her mother would retreat to their own room immediately following dinner. The tension and hostility was almost never directly expressed; however, there were frequent snide remarks. The grandmother served as a pivotal person in the communication system. Lana's mother would talk to the grandmother, and the aunt would talk to the grandmother, but rarely would they talk to each other. Lana's mother always served the role of victim. Lana states that her mother was extremely sensitive to her grandmother's criticism of her, and her grandmother was constantly criticizing her for the way she raised Lana, as well as for other things. When Lana was in her second year of high school, the situation got so intolerable that Lana and her mother moved out of the house and got an apartment about a mile away.

Lana states that she did not get along well with her cousins, one of whom was two years older than she, and the other of whom was about her age. While growing up and then in "adulthood," Lana was regarded by the extended family as somewhat outside of the mainstream-for example, Lana was only the second member of her extended family, which included nine cousins, who went to college.

Lana states that even her relationship with her mother, although close and dependent in some ways, was distant when it came to showing feelings. Her mother rarely discussed how she felt about Lana's father, other men, or other members of her family. Sexuality was never talked about.

Lana's mother had one male friend who was a steady companion for more than ten years. This man would come over sometimes and watch television with her mother during Lana's high school years. Lana states that this relationship was rather stable; it never got closer or more distant. For example, the possibility of marriage was never raised.

Lana has had little contact with her father. When she was young, her father came around once in a while when he was in town. He was described by Lana as a vagabond type, driving around the country in a pickup camper, working at bars for short periods of time, never being able to save any money, and drinking quite a bit. He sometimes sent a little money to help pay for the care of Lana, but this was infrequent. Lana always wished she could know him better. On two occasions during her childhood, she went with her mother to see her father, but she only has vague memories of these trips. Toward the end of grammar school, she lost touch with him. During junior high school she began writing him again, and in high school she had a desire to get to know him better. During her senior year she visited him in Oregon. At that time he had remarried, and she spent a week with him and his wife. She was rather disappointed by the visit, because he treated her as a guest and she had hoped that the relationship would be closer. Since that visit, she has seen her father several times on visits to Oregon, with similar reactions. Her father came down from Oregon for both her college graduation and her wedding.

Lana dated her husband-to-be in high school. He was the only steady boyfriend she had before she was married. They became involved sexually while she was in high school. Sexuality was primarily of the back-seat-of-thecar variety. Lana states she was largely unsatisfied with sex at that time and felt a great deal of guilt about it.

Lana married when she completed her second year of college. She then began going to college part-time while supporting her husband through college with a job. After three years her husband graduated from college and began teaching. She returned to college and got her degree when she was twenty-four. At that time she and her husband decided to have a child, and she became pregnant. Just prior to her pregnancy, Lana's husband began to have affairs, which she did not find out about until after she was pregnant. She stated that she remained married mostly because she was afraid that she could not get along without her husband. At least in part, the pregnancy was an excuse to cling to her husband. Immediately following her husband's graduation from college, Lana and her husband bought a house, which was about three or four blocks away from Lana's mother's house. Her mother had returned to living with her own mother.

Several months after the birth of Lana's baby boy, she separated from her husband and shortly afterward filed for divorce. This was in response to her husband's affairs and her general feeling of becoming more distant from him. She saw separation from her husband, she stated, as the only way in which she could be a less dependent person. In fact, her greatest dependency had always been on her mother, from whom she had never lived more than a few blocks away; this dependency increased after the divorce, although not without ambivalence.

When Lana first came to therapy she was still living in the house within several blocks of her mother with her 2 ½ year-old child, John. Every day, prior to going to work, she took her boy over to her grandmother, who babysat him during her working hours. When she went out, she usually relied on either her mother or her grandmother to take care of her child. She stated that her relationship with her ex-husband stabilized somewhat over time in that she considered him one of her best friends but that their romantic relationship was completely over. Her husband had a new girlfriend. She saw her husband about once every two weeks, when he came over to see their child.

She enjoyed her son a great deal. She stated that sometimes she felt she depended on her boy for intimacy too much. Sometimes she felt guilty because she did not spend as much time with her boy as she felt she should. On the whole she was a good mother, showing care and concern for the boy; they appeared to have a good relationship.

Lana felt trapped by her relationship with her mother. On the one hand she desired more distance from her mother, while at the same time she feared her distance would leave her mother alone and depressed. She stated, "Mother is too dependent on me. I feel sorry for her. She is so alone. I am the only thing that she ever had." She also was quite angry at her mother, because, in her words, "Mother will not accept me for what I really am. I'm afraid to tell mother about myself because I'm afraid of her mental state. She really flips out. She is not having any fun. I always think about her when I'm having fun. . . couldn't mother be having fun doing this. I see her as pathetic. I'm the only thing she ever had." She went on to say, "She treats me like a kid. I wish my mother had confidence in me to be friends rather than always trying to tell me what to do." What Lana did not state until much later in therapy was how she also felt trapped by her own feelings of dependency upon her mother, which made her angry at herself.

Lana's relationship with her mother thus was more an adolescent's relationship than that of a twenty-nine-year-old independent adult. When Lana had first started therapy, she had just begun to make a few friends. She had one boyfriend and a few women friends. She felt ambivalent toward her boyfriend, which in many ways reflected her relationship with her mother. With both, she would frequently request greater independence while her actions would establish more dependence. For example, her boyfriend would frequently spend up to several weeks living at her house; during this time she would tell him she wanted him to move out and then would encourage him to spend the night. She would treat him badly at times and then feel guilty: "I feel like I owe him something . . . I use him all the time for security . . . I don't really know if I ever loved him." This dynamic—of feeling caught in the relationship because of needing security yet all the time wanting to break off the relationship—corresponds closely to Lana's relationship with her mother; she constantly feels as if she wants to be more distant, while needing the security provided by the relationship. The similarity also extends to the feelings of guilt that she has when she does not provide for the dependency needs of the other party.

In reviewing the variables related to the separation process, a number of adverse circumstances can be found to be affecting Lana. There also are areas of significant strength on which to build.

Variable 1. The readiness of the individual for independence. Lana is obviously able to provide for herself. She is vocationally successful. When she tries, she makes friends easily. She is a good mother. She could operate effectively if she moved away from her mother.

Variable 2. Cognitive influences. Lana's ability to understand change is well developed. She is able to find continuity of meaning in changing situations. Her abilities to identify and internalize strengths of others is also well developed.

Variable 3. The nature of the parent-child relationship. Lana was abandoned by her father, making separation from her mother more dangerous. Lana's relationship with her mother is overinvolved and maintained by fear and guilt. The whole family is anger-inhibited, making the open discussion of disagreements difficult, again limiting self-definition, that is, independence. To achieve greater separation, Lana will have to develop a greater ability to tolerate guilt or not feel so guilty about separating, or her mother will have to cease giving guilt signals when Lana moves toward separation.

Variable 4. The past experiences of the parents and the adolescent in separation. Lana has had poor separation experiences. Her mother has not been a good role model in her relationship with her own mother. Separation has felt like rejection. Her father abandoned her mother, and Lana's mother has made it clear that she would feel rejected if Lana separated from her. For Lana to separate, she must view separation in a new way.

Variable 5. Cultural influences. Living in the San Francisco Bay area Lana has received strong support from her peers to move toward separation from her parents. However, such a diverse culture has made the search for an integrated identity separate from her mother's a more difficult process.

Initially in psychotherapy, Lana talked most about issues related to the early stages of the separation process. For example, she had an opportunity to go camping with a friend, which she had wanted to do for a long time, but she was angry at herself because it made her nervous to think about staying away from home. She felt split from herself, unable to decide on future plans. Issues related to an identity diffusion were discussed; for example, she went to a dress shop and was not able to decide on the style of dress that she felt fit her present view of herself. She avoided being alone and felt very dependent on her new friends. This dependency made her angry with herself. She wanted to move from her home to a new location but felt that she could not give up the security.

Lana's initial response to me as a therapist was to try to please me. She felt insecure in her relationship with me, feeling as though she had to be a good patient or else she would be rejected. Therefore she avoided all conflict and discussed things she felt the therapist would like to hear. Her tactics indicated her dependency on my view of her and her feeling of needing someone. The initial goal, then, was to help her talk freely about what she was interested in, giving her the message that she would not be rejected if she disagreed or even became angry with me, thus creating less dependency on my view of her.

The message that I was trying to get across to her was that her independence from me would be accepted without her having to feel guilty. She was also to know that she was expected to take a share of the responsibility for directing the therapeutic process. Encouraging one to be independent is of course a paradox. In this situation, it was a therapeutic paradox, in that it communicated to Lana an acceptance of both dependency and independence. This is a message that good parents give their children and that good therapists give their patients. Of course it cannot be given unless one really feels it.

We avoided discussing Lana's weaknesses and, rather, concentrated on where she showed strength and ability in her interpersonal interactions with me and on how these would serve her productively in her interactions with others. Over a period of two months she became increasingly comfortable in openly discussing issues. It was the first time she had ever talked about many of these issues, such as becoming angry, having sexual feelings toward particular people, and feeling depressed.

Not long afterwards, she began talking to some of her close friends about these issues. She also began to experiment in her relationships on a number of different fronts. For example, she began to date new men and found this exciting, although in some cases scary. This raised questions within her regarding morality. She had resolved the issue of having an affair with her boyfriend, but she was uncertain about having sex with men with whom she had had shorter-term relationships. She went on to have sexual affairs with two different men over a period of several months. She felt ambivalent about these affairs. She felt guilty and wondered what this meant in terms of her identity. The prominent meaning of these affairs to her was that she did not have to be dependent on one individual-that she was capable of making new acquaintances and of being interesting to people in a wide variety of ways. Another more unconscious meaning was that she was not bound to her mother's morality but that she should make these decisions on her own. Initially she could not decide if she felt guilt over these affairs because she disapproved or because her mother disapproved. She stopped having affairs when she decided that they were not right for her. Prior to this, however, she attempted to get the therapist to resolve the problem. The therapist maintained the stance that he thought that she knew best how to respond to her own needs, both sexual and moral.

On the whole, Lana felt good about making new friends, both with men and with women, enhancing her self-esteem. For the first time she was having a good experience in proving her independence to herself and to others. Her most important authority figure, her psychotherapist, did not try to make her feel guilty for this as others had in the past but, rather, comfortably accepted her and attempted to communicate this to her.

Lana became more critical of me and our interaction. For example, she stated that she was quite angry at me for an interpretation that I had made the week before. She felt that my interpretation was wrong and that she had a much better idea about what was going on; she felt misunderstood. In listening to her view, I realized that it was a superior interpretation. I said so, giving her the message that she was able to make interpretations that were equal or superior to mine. She accepted this ambivalently, as teenagers are ambivalent about seeing the flaws of their parents. On the one hand they realize the opportunity for self-reliance, while at the same time they are uncomfortable with the responsibility.

During this period Lana talked a great deal about change. Nearly every week she talked about either wanting to take a trip or wanting to move. She also talked about wanting to stop psychotherapy. She stated, "At the beginning of therapy I felt a need to come, but now I feel more secure in myself. I don't really need to come anymore. I got mad at myself for not following through and stopping therapy." This was an ambivalent feeling. She also remained somewhat dependent and afraid of change. She said, "I used to get scared when I went from junior high school to high school to college, but once there, I adapted. But I'm afraid to change." She went on to say, "I feel upset about the impulse to quit, but I don't know why. I enjoy talking to someone objective, but I feel as though I no longer really need to." Following her openness regarding her feelings about our relationship, she would frequently feel guilty and attempt to undo what she had said. I would take care not to communicate rejection, while agreeing with her view of her growing independence. This was possible because she was in fact much more confident in herself and had become more independent.

What Lana expected in these interactions was for the therapist to tell her directly or indirectly that she really needed therapy and that her desire for termination was premature. This would have corresponded to her relationships with her mother, her boyfriend, and her husband, who, because of their dependence on Lana, would first let her know how much she needed them and then let her know how much they needed her. This message was primarily covert, and Lana would respond by feeling guilty. However, she would also get some safety from her own ambivalence concerning separation.

When the notion was brought up of setting an approximate time for termination and working toward it, she told me that she was not ready to set a date. This interaction established that, as with other aspects of our therapeutic process, she had a share of the responsibility and control. This response also openly brought to the therapeutic process her ambivalence toward separation.

After this session Lana discussed terminating therapy nearly every week. This again served as a model for her relationship with others. She began talking to her boyfriend openly about wanting to break off the relationship. Around this time Lana started her three-year-old child in nursery school. Thus, she avoided bringing her child to her grandmother's house and stopped seeing her mother more than once or twice a week.

After many sessions in which she discussed a desire and a fear of going to Hawaii for a vacation, she followed through on this desire. However, her ambivalence concerning separation was still evident. She stated, "When I decided to go, I felt elated. I immediately went down and made reservations. However, once the reservations were made, the rest of the day I felt almost continuously as if I were going to cry."

Following her two-week trip to Hawaii, she had a significant uplift in mood, talked more about moving, and told her boyfriend that she no longer wanted him to stay with her. This time the message was clear, and he moved out. Her statements about terminating therapy became stronger. The week after coming back she said, "I guess I should think about stopping therapy. Traveling gave me strength. I feel much better."

During this period, approximately eight months after therapy had begun, Lana had frequent mood swings. She would feel good after making a move toward independence and then feel sadness at recognizing her separateness from others. She was clearly dealing with the issues of the affective response to separation, the third stage. Rather than seeing these sad periods as a problem, the therapist supported her strength at recognizing what she had to give up to become more independent. Handling sadness well meant strength, not illness.

At the beginning of summer she stated that she wanted to set a time to stop therapy, and the time was set for the end of summer. She said that summer is a time for change, that she felt she was going to make some changes to become independent and to move from her present location. During this period she became highly critical of me. I responded to her criticism by explaining the reasons for my viewpoint and by accepting the fact that we could think differently about issues. I avoided interpreting her criticism as a goal toward independence because I felt that this would attenuate the usefulness of the arguments. An interpretation at this point would have given the message that her arguing and disagreeing was a problem, when, in fact, they were positive forms of definition and separation.

Once again the therapeutic relationship served as a model for movement toward greater independence in other relationships. Lana began to argue with her mother and to point out their differences. She began to exhibit anger at her mother's controlling behavior, first in our discussions and later directly with her mother. Lana was still bothered, however, by fears that her mother was weak and needed her. She was also more open to confronting these feelings. I interpreted her mother's guilt-provoking behavior as very controlling and therefore not a sign of weakness but a sign of strength. We further explored other examples of her behavior that indicated that she was strong and therefore could take care of herself. I told Lana that it would be very difficult for her and her mother to become more independent from each other but that the more independent she became, the more independent her mother would become. This interpretation of her behavior set a up a situation that defined both Lana's dependent and independent behavior as positive, that is, non-guilt- provoking. This redefinition of her behavior set up a therapeutic paradox: no matter how Lana responded to her relationship, it was acceptable. Haley (1976) provides a detailed discussion of therapeutic paradox.

In Hawaii Lana had spent her time with a man whom she was interested in and vice versa. She had, however, responded to his letters ambivalently because she feared she might become involved with him and would lose her new-found independence. Two weeks following the session just discussed, she was more confident in her independence and responded positively to his suggestion of visiting her. At this point Lana decided that she desired to remarry and move further away from her mother. As she felt more confident in her independence, she also felt more comfortable with closeness. During these sessions, the therapist became significantly less active making almost no suggestions or interpretations but primarily being supportive. The message that I was trying to convey was that I saw her as less dependent on therapy. She recognized this and mentioned on several occasions, "It seems as though you don't have as much to say as you had in the past. I guess I'm pretty much doing it for myself," with which I immediately agreed.

At the end of summer Lana resigned from her teaching duties and flew to Hawaii to live with Jack. Six months later I received a letter from her stating that she had been living with Jack, and while she occasionally felt bad about her mother, on the whole she was delighted with her lifestyle. She and Jack were considering getting married in the near future.

By following this case history one can see that the therapeutic relationship was primarily an experience of moving from dependence to greater independence. Lana was first able to be more independent within the relationship. As these things were occurring within therapy, they were also occurring with her close friends and then with her mother. This led to her ultimate separation from her mother in a healthy, developmental way.

In the final stages of the therapeutic process, as Lana had become more separate, she used identification to feel independent. As the separation process would not really be complete until she actually moved away, it was expected that the identification process would continue. This identification was cultivated by a tacit permission throughout the therapeutic process-that is, looking positively at what she was able to do for herself, which was what the therapist had previously done. The therapist must take care to allow identification to occur without overtly encouraging it, as this would be seen as a form of control.

In many respects this process reflects the usual process of adolescentparental separation. As has been stated, the peer group and/or mentor serves many of the functions of the therapist in the usual process. Nonpsychotherapists can be helpful to people who are stuck in the separation process. Teachers have been seen to be very therapeutic, often without their even being aware of it. They have provided many of the experiences that occur in the therapeutic process. However, this does not commonly happen; people who are troubled by separation usually choose relationships with people who encourage dependence rather than independence. Another common problem is the encouraging of independence at too rapid a pace, which ultimately fails. Any process is therapeutic in helping resolve separation issues if it reflects the natural process of separation.

As in any interpersonal relationship such as psychotherapy, the interactions that occur are so complex that any attempt at describing them is, on some levels, ridiculously reductionistic and simplistic. If this is understood, however, it does not mean that such descriptions are useless. The preceding descriptions of helping people through the separation process have helped me to be successful in helping others. It is hoped that these accounts will be useful to others as well.

References

Alvarez, A. *The Savage God: A Study of Suicide.* New York: Random House, 1971.

Averill, J. R. "Grief: Its Nature and Significance." *Psychological Bulletin,* Vol. 70, No. 6, 1968, pp. 721-748.

Baittle, B., and Offer, D. "On the Nature of Male Adolescent Rebellion." *Adolescent Psychiatry, Volume I: Developmental and Clinical Studies.* New York: Basic Books, 1971.

Bateson, G. et al. *Steps to an Ecology of Mind.* New York: Ballantine,

1975. Benedict, R. *Patterns of Culture.* New York: Houghton Mifflin,
Bloom, M., Ralph, N., and Freedman, M. "Patterns of Faculty Response to Growing Student
1961. Diversity." *New Directions for Higher Education: Facilitating Faculty Development,* 4 (1),1973.

Bios, P. *On Adolescence: A Psychoanalytic Interpretation.* New York: The Free Press of Glencoe, 1962.

____. "The Second Individuation Process of Adolescence." A. H. Esman (Editor). *The Psychology of Adolescence.* New York: International Universities Press, 1975.

Bowlby, J. *Attachment and Loss. Volume 1, Attachment.* New York: Basic Books,

1969. ____. *Attachment and Loss. Volume 2, Separation.* New York: Basic Books,
____. "Childhood Mourning and its Implications for Psychiatry." *American Journal of Psychiatry,*
1973.   1961, p. 118, 481.

____. "The Making and Breaking of Affectional Bonds." *British Journal of Psychiatry,* 130, 1977, pp.
            201-210.
Bradley, S. "The Relationship of Early Maternal Separation to Borderline Personality in Children

and Adolescents: A Pilot Study." *American Journal of Psychiatry*, 136, April 1979, p. 4 A.

Breger, L. *From Instinct to Identity: The Development of Personality.* Englewood Cliffs, N.J.: Prentice-Hall, 1974.

Burham, D. L. "The Special Problem Patient: Victim or Agent of Splitting?" *Psychiatry: Journal for the Study of Interpersonal Process, 29*, 1966, p. 2.

Darwin, C. *On the Origin of the Species by Means of Natural Selection.* London: John Murray,

1859. ____. *The Expression of Emotions in Man and Animals.* London: John Murray, 1872.
Deutsch, H. "Some Forms of Emotional Distrubance and Their Relationship to Schizophrenia." *Psychoanalytic Quarterly,* 1942, p. 11, 301.

Eibl-Eibesfeldt, I. *Ethology: The Biology of Behavior.* New York: Holt, Rinehart, and Winston, 1970.

Edelson, M. "Termination of Intensive Psychotherapy." Thomas, C. C. (Editor). *American Lectures in Psychiatry.* Washington, D.C.: American Psychiatric Association, 1963.

Erikson, E. H. *Childhood and Society.* New York: Norton,

1950. ____. *Identity: Youth and Crisis.* New York: Norton,
____. "The Concept of Ego Identity." *The Journal of the American Psychoanalytic Association,* 1956, 1968.   p. 4, 56.

____. "Reflections on the Life Cycle of Doctor Borge." *Daedalus.* Spring, 1976.

Fierman, L. B. (Editor). *Effective Psychotherapy: The Contribution of Hellmuth Kaiser.* New York: The Free Press, 1965.

Freud, S. (1921) "Ego and the Id." *Standard Edition.* 19:12-66. London: Hogarth Press, 1961. ____.

(1917) "Mourning and Melancholia." *Standard Edition.* 14:243-260. London: Hogarth Press,

1957.

____. (1932) "New Introductory Lectures on Psychoanalysis." *Standard Edition.* 22:5-182. London: Hogarth Press, 1964.

Ginott, H. G. *Between Parent and Teenager.* New York: Macmillan Co.,

1969. Goodall (van Lawick) J. *In the Shadow of Man.* New York: Dell, 1971.
____. "The Behavior of Free-Living Chimpanzees in the Gombe Stream Area." *Animal Behavior Monographs,* 1 (3), 1968.

____. and Hamburg, D. A. "Chimpanzee Behavior as a Model for the Behavior of Early Man: New Evidence on Possible Origins of Human Behavior." Arieti, (Editor). *American Handbook of Psychiatry, Volume 6.* New York: Basic Books, 1975.

Grinker, R., Werble, B., and Drye, R. *The Borderline Syndrome.* New York: Basic Books, 1968.

Gunderson, J. G., Carpenter, W. T., and Strauss, J. S. "Borderline and Schizophrenic Patients." *American Journal of Psychiatry,* 132, 1975, p. 12.

Gunderson, J. G., and Singer, M. "Defining Borderline Patients: An Overview." *American Journal of Psychiatry,* 132, January 1975, p. 1.

Haley, J. *Problem-Solving Therapy.* New York: Harper and Row,

1976. ____. *Uncommon Therapy.* New York: Norton, 1973.

Hass, H. *The Human Animal.* New York: Dell, 1972. Hinde, R.

A. *Animal Behavior.* New York: McGraw-Hill, 1966.
Hollingsworth, L. S. *The Psychology of the Adolescent.* New York: Appleton and Century, 1928.

Kaiser, H. *Effective Psychotherapy: The Contribution of Hellmuth Kaiser.* Fierman, L. B. (Editor). New York: The Free Press, 1965.

Kernberg, O. "Borderline Personality Organization." *Journal of the American Psychoanalytic Association,* 15, 1967, p. 641.

Knight, R. "Borderline States." *Bulletin of the Menninger Clinic,* 17, 1953, p. 1. Langs, R. *The Technique of Psychoanalytic Psychotherapy, Volume 2.* New York: Aronson, 1974.

Levinson, D. et al. "The Psychosocial Development of Men in Early Adulthood and the Mid-Life Transition." Roff, M. and Ricks, D. F. (Editors). *Life History Research in Psychopathology.* Minneapolis: University of Minnesota Press, 1970.

Lewis, C. S. *A Grief Observed.* New York: Seabury Press, 1961.

Lorenz, K. *Evolution and Modification of Behavior.* Chicago: University of Chicago Press, 1965.

____. "The Enmity Between the Generations and Its Probable Ethological Causes." M. W. Piers (Editor). *Play and Development.* New York: Norton, 1972.

Lowenthal, M. F. and Chiriboga, D. "Transition to the Empty Nest." *Archives of General Psychiatry,* 26, 1976.

Lowenthal, M. F., Chiriboga, D., and Turner, M. *Four Stage of Life: A Comparative Study of Women and Men Facing Transitions.* San Francisco: Jossey-Bass, 1975.

Mahler, M. S. *On Symbiosis and the Vicissitudes of Individuation.* New York: International Universities Press, 1968.

Mahler, M. S., Pine, F., and Bergman, A. *The Psychological Birth of the Human Infant.* New York: Basic Books, 1975.

Marris, P. *Loss and Change.* New York: Pantheon Books, 1974.

Masterson, J. F. *Psychotherapy of the Borderline Adult-A Developmental Approach.* New York: Brunner/Mazel, 1976.

____. "The Psychiatric Significance of Adolescent Turmoil." *American Journal of Psychiatry,* 124,

1968, p. 11.

_____. *Treatment of the Borderline Adolescent: A Developmental Approach.* New York: Wiley Interscience, 1972.

Mead, M. *Coming of Age in Samoa.* New York: William Morrow,

1928. _____. *Growing Up in New Guinea.* New York: William Morrow,

1930. Morris, D. *The Naked Ape.* New York: McGraw-Hill, 1967.

Mueller, P. S. and Orfanidis, M. M. "A Method of Co-Therapy for Schizophrenic Families." *Family Process,* Vol. 15, No. 2 (June), 1976, pp. 179-191.

Muensterberger, W. "The Adolescent in Society." A. H. Esman (Editor). *The Psychology of Adolescence.* New York: International Universities Press, 1975.

Murphy, E. B. et al. *Development of Autonomy and Parent-Child Interaction in Late Adolescence.* Maryland: National Institute of Mental Health, 1962.

Murray, H. A. *Explorations in Personality.* New York: Oxford University Press, 1938.

Napier, J. R. *The Roots of Mankind.* Washington: Smithsonian, 1970. Offer, D. *The*

Psychological World of the Teenager. New York: Basic Books, 1969. Offer, D. and Offer,

J. B. *From Teenage to Young Manhood.* New York: Basic Books, 1975.

Oremland, J. "Three Hippies: A Study of Late-Adolescent Identity Formation." *International Journal of Psychoanalytic Psychotherapy,* 1974.

Paris, J. "The Oedipus Complex-A Critical Re-Examination." *Canadian Psychiatric Association Journal,* Vol. 21, 1976, pp. 173-179.

Parkes, L. M. *Bereavement: Studies of Grief in Adult Life.* New York: International Universities Press, 1972.

Peskin, H. Personal Communications, 1977.

Pfeiffer, E. "Borderline States." *Disorders of the Nervous System,* 35, 1974, p. 212.

Piaget, J. "The Intellectual Development of the Adolescent." A. H. Esman (Editor). *The Psychology of Adolescence.* New York: International Universities Press, 1975.

Piaget, J. and Inhelder, B. *The Psychology of the Child.* New York: Basic Books, 1969. Rank,

O. *The Trauma of Birth.* New York: Harper and Row, 1973. ____. *Will Therapy and Truth and Reality.* New York: Alfred A. Knopf, 1945. Sanford, N. Lectures on Self and Society at

The Wright Institute, Berkeley, California, 1970. ____. *Self and Society.* New York:

Atherton, 1967.

Scagnelli, J. "Hypnotherapy with Schizophrenic and Borderline Patients: Summary of Therapy with Eight Patients." *The American Journal of Clinical Hypnosis,* Vol. 19, No. 1 (July), 1976, pp. 33-38.

Schoenberg, B. et al. (Editors). *Bereavement: Its Psychosocial Aspects.* New York: Columbia University Press, 1975.

Singer, M. Grand Rounds Presentation. Department of Psychological and Social Medicine. San Francisco, Calif.: Pacific Medical Center, 1976.

Stebbins, G. L. *Processes of Organic Evolution.* Englewood Cliffs, N.J.: Prentice-Hall, 1966.

Stierlin, H., Levi, L. D., and Savord, R. J. "Parental Perceptions of Separating Children." *Family Process,* 1971, p. 10, 411.

Stierlin, H. *Separating Parents and Adolescents.* New York: Quadrangle,

1974. Sullivan, H. *Conceptions of Modem Psychiatry.* New York: Norton,

1940.

_____. *The Interpersonal Theory of Psychiatry.* New York: Norton, 1953.

Washburn, S. L. *The Study of Human Evolution.* Eugene, Ore.: University of Oregon Press, 1968.

Washburn, S. L. and Moore, R. *Ape to Man: A Study of Human Evolution.* New York: Little, 1974.

Washburn, S. L. and Lancaster, C. S. "The Evolution of Hunting." Dolhi- now, P. and Sarich, V. M. (Editors). *Background for Man.* Boston: Little, Brown, 1971.

Watzlawick, P. *The Language of Change.* New York: Basic Books, 1978.

Weiss, R. S. *Marital Separation.* New York: Basic Books, 1975.

Wiener, N. *Cybernetics: Or Control and Communication in the Animal and Machine.* Cambridge, Mass.: M.I.T. Press, 1948.

Notes

[1] For a touching autobiographical account of this process, see C. S. Lewis's *A Grief Observed*, 1961.

[2] All subjects' names, as well as minor details, have been changed to protect the anonymity of the subjects.

www.ingramcontent.com/pod-product-compliance
Lightning Source LLC
Chambersburg PA
CBHW051856170526
45168CB00001B/132